MW01717458

Million Americans Dead

A 2020 Pandemic Journal

Janet Farrington Graham

ANGELKEEP PUBLISHING

A Million Americans Dead
A 2020 Pandemic Journal

Angelkeep Publishing

ISBN: 979-8-9904518-6-5 (print)
ISBN: 979-8-9904518-7-2 (ePub)

Note to the reader: This journal is a personal account of two pandemic years, 2020-2022. I have verified information with as much accuracy as a non-journalist can muster using a dozen sources of information, sometimes daily. However, this journal should not be used as a primary source; it is not intended to be scholarly or scientific. I have written this journal so those who lived through the pandemic can remember, and so those who come after will understand how more than a million Americans perished in the 2020 pandemic. JFG, August 2024.

AI cover image generated by Adobe Firefly
Cover and interior design: Syrp & Co.

Angelkeep Publishing

So our grandchildren will know

Contents

Introduction

My husband and I still live in the log cabin on the edge of the Oregon wilderness where we raised our three children. They are grown and pursuing careers in two metro areas: Michael and Rachel in Denver, and Hannah in Portland. Keith and I retired from medicine and mental health in 2019.

We were in Hawaii when reports of the Coronavirus first aired on national news. In January 2020, China reported 139 cases and 38 dead in Wuhan. The WHO initially said not to worry, "There is no human-to-human transmission."

By the time we returned home on February 4, several cruise ships were under quarantine due to new cases and the US restricted most air travel from China. On February 26, 2020, a cluster was discovered in a Kirkland, Washington nursing home and thirty days later there were 85,000 cases with nearly 1,300 dead in the US.

As a writer and counselor, I document the challenges of family life through narrative journals when major events move me. During a walk in the woods on March 11, 2020, I pondered what effect a global pandemic would have on the world, how those not yet born might be impacted, what my grandchildren would learn about the pandemic decades later. I decided to write.

The virus thrives on weakness and America was quickly exposed. We were shockingly unprepared for a health emergency. There were never enough test kits or protective gear or medicines or machines or morgues. Even basic mitigation efforts were increasingly ineffective once President Trump politicized the pandemic for re-election purposes and used anti-science as a loyalty pledge for his base. The virus became a hoax...and a weapon.

We also did not anticipate a sudden public response to racial injustice. We were appalled when a White policeman kneeled on the neck of a Black man for nine minutes and twenty-nine seconds, killing him without cause, and then encouraged when tens of millions—here and abroad—began a sustained call for justice.

Could we have known that the peaceful transfer of presidential power in 2021 would be threatened by an assault upon the US Capitol aired in real time around the world? Or that miles of barbed wire and thousands of troops would circle those same steps during the inauguration of our 46th president just two weeks later?

We expected hurricanes and floods and wildfires and ice storms and earthquakes and tsunamis and volcanic eruptions and plagues of locust, but the intensity of these climate events took most of us by surprise. As did the anger and aggression and misinformation about the pandemic that caused so much unnecessary illness and death.

This journal begins with lockdowns and mandates and moves through economic and social and political upheaval and ends two years later with over a million Americans dead and a handful of ideas about power and progress, wealth and inequality, false liberty and true freedom. This journal ends with a message to the world from Ukraine: Democracy is worth defending with your life.

I hope all our grandchildren benefit from reading this journal. The millions who are dead from COVID might be a cautionary tale, but the numbers say nothing of the real suffering; only a witness can do that.

Part One:
The First Wave

March 11-August 10, 2020

MARCH 11, 2020

Due to a strange "new" virus—Coronavirus—a state of emergency was just issued in Oregon and Colorado and a few other states; social distancing has been recommended to slow the spread. Residents are advised to wash hands, limit gatherings, and stand six feet apart. Hugs and handshakes are strongly discouraged.

The Center for Disease Control (CDC) has failed to provide adequate testing, so the number of cases reported in the US represents a small percentage of probable infections. As of today, there are 118,000 cases reported worldwide and 4,300 deaths in fifty-four countries which will likely double in a week.

The National Basketball Association (NBA) suspended the 2020 season after several players tested positive for the virus, and then the US restricted travel from Europe, which sent vacationers and expats to the airports in a rush. When they arrived at JFK and O'Hare, thousands were crowded together in queues because the US government neglected to prepare for their homecoming. There was no "social distancing" going on at US airports over the weekend and no masks—just panic.

I have asked the kids to stock up on essentials and they sound frustrated by my "apocalyptic talk," but I have a very bad feeling about this.

MARCH 15, 2020

	Cases	Deaths
World:	**169,511**	**6,520**
US:	**3,485**	**65**

After downplaying the risk from the virus for the past two months, President Trump finally declared a national emergency which frees up resources for the states. Washington State—where the first case appeared in the US on January 21—had the most cases during the past month but New York quickly caught up after one lawyer infected nearly fifty people at a conference. New York has 700 cases, but the schools remain open along with the restaurants and bars.

The CDC has recommended there be no gatherings over fifty people in the nation, and Oregon has closed K-12 schools until April. Colleges have followed suit and Rachel has 1,200 classes at Metropolitan State University (MSU) in Denver to bring online as part of her job as an online course developer. She has great job security and incredible stress.

Michael's two coffee shops—Lost City Denver and Lost City Capitol Hill—will not open tomorrow due to a "take-out only" order from the mayor for all restaurants and bars in the city; there will be no dining in and no one is walking by.

MARCH 16, 2020

Today is Hannah's 27th birthday and she celebrated by going to a few bars in downtown Portland on Saturday night. She lives with two girlfriends who also have boyfriends, so it is difficult for these millennials to socially distance as well as their parents would hope. We console ourselves with the widely held belief that the virus mainly threatens the elderly who have chronic health issues.

Michael opened his second coffee shop across from the Colorado Capitol building just thirty-nine days ago but now most of his customers are either newly unemployed or working from home. He spent the weekend retooling Lost City Capitol Hill to facilitate the preparation and delivery of free meals to people in need throughout the Denver area. His 15,000 square foot industrial kitchen, included in his lease, is now the hub for the Denver Metro Emergency Food Network (DMEFN), a new collaboration between non-profit organizations and several for-profit delivery groups.

MARCH 19, 2020

California has become the first state to issue "stay-at-home" orders that extend to all non-essential businesses and residents. Many states have closed schools and issued take-out-only orders for restaurants and bars.

Italy has reported 41,000 cases and 5,000 deaths, overtaking China as the world's hotspot, and Europe is in full lockdown. China reports no new cases after ten weeks of aggressive containment, which gives the rest of the world hope…and raises suspicion. Unfortunately, few places have been able to lockdown citizens as easily or test for the virus as widely as this communist country.

In the future, historians might figure out why China silenced their own doctors who discovered the disease in late 2019 and then reported to the World Health Organization that there was no human-to-human transmission. The world continued traveling to and from China, quickly spreading the virus around the globe.

The Denver Metro Emergency Food Network (DMEFN) raised $8,000 in 24 hours and delivered their first 128 meals.

MARCH 20, 2020

The week began with the largest one day drop in stock market history: 2,997 points in a single day. There have been mass business closings, layoffs, and public-school closings. The week ended with the worst stock market loss since the 2008 crash, with the DOW losing 17.3% of its value.

The US has one of the lowest per capita testing rates in the world due to the failure of the CDC to provide accurate tests. People are flooding hospitals and clinics with requests for tests but the few they have are unreliable. President Trump assures the American people in his now daily briefings that there are "millions of tests" available; he lies, frequently.

The asymptomatic nature of the disease—which can be as high as 50%—adds to the fear that the virus is spreading at alarming rates in American cities.

MARCH 22, 2020

Louisiana joined nine states—including Oregon—to issue "stay-at-home" orders to all but essential personnel and businesses to help control the spread of the virus. New Orleans allowed Mardi Gras to go forward in February and now the city has the fastest growing infection rate in the country.

Tony Spell, a pastor in Baton Rouge, decided the lockdown order was a politically motivated attempt to make President Trump look bad, so he held services as planned for over a thousand souls who crowded into his church to pray for healing. He provided bus transportation for free.

He was not the only religious leader to ignore pleas from public health officials who warned that suffering and death might descend upon those who stand too closely together...especially when singing.

Hundreds of churches held services as usual, mostly in the southern states. Hopefully, the virus will pass right over President Trump's pious supporters in the south.

The Denver Metro Emergency Food Network delivered 1,500 meals at the end of their first week.

MARCH 23, 2020

In eight days, virus infections in New York state increased to 20,000 from 700 including 157 deaths, representing nearly half of all US infections. On March 18, the governor announced there would be no stay-at-home order for New York City but changed his mind two days later. Now, one of the most densely populated cities in the country is shut down for everyone except essential workers.

Unfortunately, there are not enough ventilators or beds to care for the thousands in New York who are expected to become severely ill in the next two weeks, so the governor has been calmly and urgently pleading for help every afternoon on national television. FEMA opened four temporary medical facilities which added 1,000 beds.

Oregon's mandatory stay-at-home order went into effect today. As a medical assistant in a fertility clinic, Hannah's job may be considered non-essential, but for now the clinic will continue caring for women who have started the in-vitro process. The clinic fired half the staff and reduced Hannah's hours by 40%.

Although retired, Keith is still the public health director for Union County and is on the phone for briefings several mornings a week.

MARCH 25, 2020

Congress approved and the president signed a two trillion-dollar stimulus package called the Personal Protection Program (PPP) that includes up to $1,200 in one-time payments to most Americans, and billions in forgivable loans for small businesses who keep or rehire staff when the stay-at-home orders are lifted. President Trump refuses to issue a national order to stay at home, fearing the economic and political consequences of being the bearer of such bad news in an election year.

People congregate as usual in many of the southern states since most of the Republican governors follow the president's lead. At the most recent national briefing he spoke these encouraging words: "Wouldn't it be great if all the churches were packed on Easter Sunday? Wouldn't that be a beautiful thing?" Democrats outweigh Republicans nearly two to one in their caution regarding the virus which has quickly become politicized.

It is predicted that more than two million new unemployment claims will be filed this week, breaking all previous records, but the number could be much higher according to leading economists. There is talk of a current recession and/or global depression in the coming months. Developing countries with weak economies and few reserves will not fare well. Most countries in the world have people in the hospital with the virus which is now called COVID-19, or COVID for short.

MARCH 26, 2020

There is an unprecedented amount of baking going on in lockdown and I am no exception. After tasting a fresh batch of cinnamon rolls, my sister-in-law jokingly offered me $5 a roll to bake more, and that was all the incentive needed to make dozens. Today Keith and I made several "porch deliveries" which is a great way to touch base with housebound friends. All over the country people are ordering flour from Amazon in fifty-pound bags and baking for neighbors.

Unemployment figures for last week were released today despite a suggestion from the president that politicians hide the figures to avoid a panic. The states declined and it appears 3.3 million Americans lost their jobs last week and applied for benefits, the largest figure since the Great Depression. April rent is due in three days and there is no comprehensive forbearance in the works. Several states, Oregon included, have issued "no eviction" orders but rent strikes are still expected.

MARCH 27, 2020

My first thought upon waking up this morning was that one of our children in Denver could be infected with the virus, given Michael's meal delivery service and his regular contact with Rachel and her fiancé, Kevin, who live two city blocks away. I called Rachel and asked about her medical supplies, which consisted of a spray bottle of disinfectant and a small hand sanitizer.

"Will you be taking care of Kevin or Michael if they get the virus?" I asked. "Of course," she answered which means they need a home COVID care kit. Half our supplies are going to Denver.

After President Trump dismissed the virus so quickly, the country was unprepared when infections increased at an exponential rate. In late February there were fifteen cases at a retirement home in Washington State, and during a national press briefing we were told those cases would disappear; that we would beat the virus due to our excellent government response.

Four weeks later there are over 100,000 cases, very little testing, no production of supplies needed by medical workers, and no ventilators for the seriously ill. Day after day the president contradicts public health professionals—including Dr. Fauci, Director of the National Institute of Allergy and Infectious Disease (NIAID), who is our new national hero—and exaggerates the resources that are available. The governors are forced to compete to buy supplies while hundreds of Americans die. There are no price controls and no toilet paper in most cities.

Since there are so few N95 masks available, we feel guilty sending the ones from our workshop to our children or wearing them ourselves. "You don't need them," the surgeon general announced during a national press event. Right. Sure. Three N95 masks are going to Denver.

MARCH 28, 2020

	CASES	DEATHS
WORLD:	663,127	30, 861
US:	122,653	2,220

Rachel's medical box contains a big tub of disinfectant wipes, disposable gloves, a thermometer, hand sanitizer, chicken soup, dark chocolate, and three masks. When I called to see if she needed anything else, she sheepishly mentioned that there is no toilet paper in her local stores. "The shelves are empty, like in a disaster movie," she said. I am going to need a bigger box.

Wallowa County has no COVID cases yet, but we are closed like the big cities. Our three local grocery stores still have supplies, but there is no toilet paper here either. Some people only keep one or two extra rolls around so the prospect of being home all day without this necessity sent people into a panic, a good reminder of how much time we usually spend away from home, in other bathrooms.

The Denver Metro Emergency Food Network delivered 5,000 meals this week.

APRIL 3, 2020

The CDC finally told us to wear masks in all public spaces. Rachel is making hers from folded cloth, coffee filters and rubber bands, using a pattern published online; I am using Egyptian cotton pillowcases since the weave is so fine.

We do have some unexpected, good news: The world's air pollution problem has improved dramatically in the past few weeks. Gas prices are way down, and some car insurance companies are refunding a portion of monthly premiums since so few people are driving. No driving, no accidents.

There was an earthquake in Idaho this week which shook my recliner back and forth while I was watching a volcano erupt in the movie *Dante's Peak*. A snowstorm was raging outside—dropping sixteen inches—and of course there is the pandemic. "The Four Horsemen of the Apocalypse," I joked to the kids on the family message board.

The bad news is that there are over a million cases of COVID worldwide, ten million jobs lost in the US, and thousands of dead in New York City where medical staff lack personal protection equipment (PPE) and enough ventilators to keep the sick people breathing.

Hospitals barracks are being assembled in Central Park. Initially, they planned to dig trenches for the dead in Strawberry Field, but a nearby island will be used instead. Gravediggers will carve long burial trenches on Hart Island where the unknown dead have always been interned. People are not allowed to visit hospitals, so loved ones die alone and are buried alone.

Denver Emergency Food Network has delivered 15,000 meals so far.

APRIL 4, 2020

Oregon Governor Kate Brown has answered the anguish cry from New York Governor Andrew Cuomo, who pleaded for ventilators and promised to return the favor once the surge in New York has passed. He suggested that supplies follow the surge in every state where the need is greatest.

Oregon shipped 140 ventilators directly to New York, bypassing the National stockpile which is being controlled by the president's son-in-law. There are approximately 160,000 ventilators in the US, with another 12,000 in the National stockpile. Unfortunately, we recently learned the ones in storage do not work due to years of neglect.

Sweden has decided to try a pandemic experiment in herd immunity: They will leave the country open for business with a few "suggestions" for social distancing. Restaurants and shops will serve customers as usual while young people stroll, ride bikes, and visit museums and galleries. Political leaders believe the country will be better served if their healthy population is quickly infected, although two thousand scientists in Sweden vehemently disagreed in an open letter to the president. There have been 374 deaths recorded in Sweden so far.

APRIL 5, 2020

Since we live in a visually stunning vacation destination in the NE corner of Oregon, the county becomes crowded with people who rent homes and hotel rooms and RV spots every summer. Some of the restaurants and bars that are now closed due to lockdown will remain permanently closed if the summer season is lost. This is also true for the museums, art galleries, boat rental business, retail stores and almost every other local business that is part of the service and tourism industry.

A recent article in the New York Times featured residents from Joseph, Oregon discussing the benefits of isolation in rural communities, and the lack of resources if the virus surges. In response, the mayor of Joseph sent a Facebook post asking visitors to stay away, we are not open for business as usual. Not yet.

This has been a challenge for vacation communities. During a normal season, visitors are welcome but during a pandemic an influx of strangers can be deadly. Keith and I have friends who wanted to drive across two states and visit here, but we lovingly asked them to stay home, please.

My good friend and mentor, Steve Dreier, died of COVID in a New York hospital today. Last month he correctly predicted that his diminished pulmonary system would not survive a COVID infection. Godspeed, my friend.

APRIL 7, 2020

Our governor was interviewed on national news and answered questions about the successful stay-at-home initiative that appears to be flattening the curve and saving lives in Oregon. State health experts expect the peak of infections around April 20, but no one really knows. Keith will join an ethics committee task force in Union County to develop a regional COVID protocol, rules that may determine who lives and who dies. Thankfully, there are only four cases in a neighboring county so far.

Although all other state and local elections have been postponed during the pandemic, Wisconsin was the exception today. The Republican state legislature hopes to re-elect a conservative supreme court justice, so they sued to force in-person elections—all the way to the US Supreme Court which granted their petition. Wisconsin Republicans know that if everyone votes, they cannot win. The usual 180 polling places were reduced to five and masked voters waited in line for hours, six feet apart, in the rain and hail—democracy at its finest.

There were 1,900 US deaths from COVID in the past 24 hours, the highest death toll in the world.

Denver Metro Emergency Food Network delivered 1,800 meals in one day.

APRIL 9, 2020

Unemployment figures were released today. There were 6.6 million additional claims last week, bringing the total to 17 million.

Lines at the food banks are miles long, while farmers in California and Florida are letting crops rot in the fields. Without workers to harvest and transport the fruits and vegetable to restaurants and grocery stores, the food distribution chain is broken. Economists continue to warn about an economic depression but the only way to make it safe for people to work is universal testing and we do not have a federal testing policy. One American dies every forty-seven seconds, and we have no way to know who is spreading the virus.

Wallowa County has its first confirmed case of COVID-19, and the local health officials briefed the county via Facebook. They report an adequate amount of PPE, but only two ventilators which means seriously ill patients will be flown to Portland.

Several weeks ago, my brother Don and his wife Linda agreed to isolate so we could socialize outside when the weather improves. It was 70 degrees today, so we ordered a pizza to go, filled a personal cooler with beverages and enjoyed an afternoon in the sun on his deck which overlooks the Wallowa mountains. Our friend Marcy walked from her nearby home to join us. It is necessary to determine which of your friends to include in your bubble; there are many friends we will not see for a while.

APRIL 10, 2020

The managing director of the International Monetary Fund, (IMF) comprised of 186 nations, published remarks on the current global financial situation. She suggests the world is facing the worst economic fallout since the Great Depression and that the developing countries will be hardest hit. She ended her comments with a quote from Victor Hugo: *"Great perils have this beauty, that they bring to light the fraternity of strangers."*

We see no evidence of this in reports from Ecuador where bodies pile up in the streets and people beg door-to-door for food to no avail; neighbors are too frightened to open their doors to an invisible foe.

We see no evidence of this in India, where millions of migrant workers who lost jobs headed home in crowded buses and trains to rural villages where family members were too frightened to welcome them home. Unfortunately, the new quarantine barracks they have erected to isolate these workers will soon become a virus hotspot due to inadequate medical resources.

It breaks the heart to behold such scenes which are happening all over the world. It is estimated that 81% of the 3.3 billion workers in the world had their workplace fully or partially closed in the past three weeks.

On a positive note, Denver Metro Emergency Food Network delivered 3,000 meals every day this week. They have opened an additional industrial kitchen since Lost City Capitol Hill is at full capacity.

APRIL 11, 2020

The US now has the distinction of having the highest death rate from COVID of any country in the world, surpassing China. The virus hit especially hard in nursing homes, veterans' homes, prisons, and churches.

All fifty states have declared a disaster for the first time in US history. Farmers are smashing eggs they cannot sell, dumping milk they cannot afford to pasteurize, and bulldozing produce by the ton. The food supply chain is completely disrupted. The largest pork producer has closed plants and warns that the meat industry cannot function with so many sick employees.

Due to long-term inequality towards minorities in this country—including lack of access to health care and remote employment options, or healthy food or clean water or testing facilities—the death rate among African American communities is 40% higher than the general population.

America does have priorities, however. After legal challenges, gun stores were allowed to remain open leading to a 41% increase in requests for background checks and long lines snaking around gun stores in nearly every community.

APRIL 12, 2020

I dug deep in the freezer and pulled out a prime rib from last Christmas and spent the day cooking an Easter dinner to leave on Marcy's porch. My brother was on delivery duty.

Marcy was widowed just four months ago and has been isolated at home—alone with her grief. We speak on the phone daily and visit at a distance once a week during dinner deliveries, but there is no substitute for hands-on comfort. There are likely tens of thousands in lockdown who are going through the same solo grieving process due to the 23,000 loved ones who have already died from COVID.

Dozens of churches across the south and middle America defied stay-at-home orders and held Easter services on Sunday. They cited the Constitution, the primacy of God over government, and some mythical protection by the "blood of Christ" as reason enough to bring people together despite evidence of high infection rates at church.

A Baton Rouge pastor, who has already been fined for defying stay-at-home orders, held a rotating service throughout the day and used twenty-seven buses to bring believers to his virus infection festival.

It is fair to wonder how these "right-to-life" religionists reconcile the danger of spreading COVID in their communities; how they advocate for the life of the unborn but ignore their own deadly behavior with friends and family. Evangelicals should resurrect some common sense.

APRIL 13, 2020

There are seven Republican governors who have still not issued stay-at-home orders, citing constitutional and political issues. President Trump refused to issue a national order, saying it was up to the states, so there are millions of Americans simply ignoring the pandemic and public health recommendations.

Even in states with orders, many people are not willing to stay home to save lives. Mixed messages from the president have confused people and politicized the issue. On January 22 Trump said, "The virus is completely under control." On February 10 he said, "It will go away in April." On February 26 he predicted cases will soon be "down to zero." There were sixty cases then and over half a million now.

The governors were told to take care of their own states and that is what most have been trying to do. Even though equipment and testing supplies are severely limited, the president assures the public during daily briefings that everything is "perfect." Of course, there is still no national testing program.

Now he wants to "reopen the country by May 1" despite warnings from public health officials that we cannot know who does and does not have the virus without testing. In a sudden reversal he now claims total authority and publicly "agonizes" over the decision to open the states.

Trump's agony is surprising given the conservative standard of states' rights and the long-held belief that opening the states would be outside a president's authority. In response to his authoritarian claim, governors on both coasts formed coalitions to consider and implement the best strategy for areas with the highest infection. President Trump tweets about mutiny and threatens to withhold resources.

APRIL 15, 2020

	Cases	Deaths
World:	2,086,332	138,474
US:	648,003	32,443

COVID infections worldwide have doubled in just two weeks—from one million to two million—and are spreading rapidly in nations with crowded cities and few supplies or public hospitals. Just to be clear, the current death toll reported in the US does not include those who die in nursing homes, veterans' homes, private homes etc.…only deaths in hospital.

We cannot stop the pandemic until there are vaccines available which will take a year or two for development, production and distribution. Since there is currently no leadership from the US government, private/public coalitions are forming to keep track of the thousands of trials for new vaccines happening in universities and private labs around the world.

In the meantime, the Florida governor declared WWE (World Wrestling Entertainment) an essential business so they can televise matches from empty arenas. This is the same leader who refused to shut down during spring break or to issue stay-at-home orders until the virus infected tens of thousands of Floridians.

Studies have shown that implementing social distancing two weeks earlier might have prevented 90% of the COVID deaths in this country. Future generations will not spare us from a brutal review of our failure as a nation and our lack of leadership in the world.

On a positive note, air quality continues to improve, and many nations have declared an immediate ceasefire for current conflicts. And in Wisconsin, the liberal candidate for the State Supreme Court won the election against the sitting conservative judge after record turnout—only the second time in state history an incumbent judge has lost a race.

APRIL 16, 2020

Unemployment figures for last week were released today and 5.5 million have been added to the rolls, bringing the total for new unemployment filings in the last four weeks to 22 million Americans.

The stimulus fund—including direct payments, small business loans, and unemployment increases—was exhausted in less than two weeks with large payments via large banks going to large corporations after their lawyers found ways to bend the rules. For some reason, the president fired the inspector general whose job it was to oversee payments; there are reports of corporations receiving tens of millions through lobbying efforts and bank favors.

There were organized protests by armed men carrying Trump MAGA (Make America Great Again) signs and confederate flags and demanding states reopened for business. They were encouraged by the president, who tells his fans on Twitter to "LIBERATE" the states led by Democratic governors.

These "patriot" protestors stood shoulder to shoulder on state Capitol steps sporting semi-automatic rifles and red caps and long beards. They are ridiculed on social media with photos titled "Dawn of the braindead," but the threat of violence by the president's followers is loud and clear.

Meanwhile, the curve is flattening in those western states with early stay-at-home orders; infection rates in the "heartland" and the southern states are still on the rise. The largest outbreaks are in the Midwest meatpacking plants that are now closing. And still, we have no federal testing program.

APRIL 17, 2020

Due to pressure from the president and his base, Jacksonville, Florida beaches have been re-opened during specific hours with strict guidelines, but people are so happy to be "free," social distancing guidelines are literally out the window.

Texas wants to be the first state to fully "reopen for business" and will loosen restrictions starting Monday. The skeptical side of my brain thinks this might be related to the presidential election in November and the battle for these two almost "purple" states. Neither state has reached its first infection peak according to epidemiologists but regardless, they are "ready."

Everyone was surprised when one northern California county began aggressively testing for antibodies and found between 50%-80%

more signs of virus than during regular testing. This virus will be impossible to contain without more testing. Imagine how many blissfully ignorant virus carriers are running around the US…and the world. "This is just the beginning," warned one Harvard epidemiologist

Last night's family Zoom chat was reassuring and uneventful. All four young adults have retained their jobs and show no signs of COVID.

The Denver Metro Emergency Food Network delivered 23,000 meals this week, bringing the total to 57,000 meals delivered since March 18, surpassing their initial goal of 50,000 meals in the first thirty days.

APRIL 18, 2020

To deflect attention from the fact the US still has no national testing program and the highest infection rate in the world, President Trump is encouraging right-wing extremists to protest the same policies he advocates during his daily briefings from the White House lawn. The chaos and confusion are designed to deflect blame and disarm the public as part of his re-election strategy. Blame the governors, blame the liberal media, blame the Chinese.

Every public health expert still believes we need more testing before we can open the states. There is some good news regarding the flattening of curves, but people assume there will be just one peak. An epidemiologist from Harvard has suggested we should imagine the virus rate as a mountain range with peaks and valleys, clusters and spikes…and some flattening of curves.

APRIL 19, 2020

The protests in the United States against stay-at-home orders are organized and encouraged by right-wing political groups, who also protests in Europe against orders to stay home.

During the past week there were protests in Mumbai by migrant workers who have no place to go, protests in Beirut against inflation which will only get worse, and unrest in Brazil where their president prides himself on making no plans to combat the virus.

The International Monetary Fund (IMF) reported that social unrest will heat up as economies fail. The outlook in developing countries does look bleak, considering their limited healthcare systems and lack of supplies. There are twelve nations in Africa that do not have a single ventilator between them.

Although there were protests in half a dozen states to end lockdown orders, 80% of Americans approve of the order. And in other polling, support for President Trump's handling of the virus dropped six points to the low 40's, which is trouble during an election year. It feels like the hesitation to criticize the president is softening among his friends and advisors, although he can easily raise a mob.

April 20, 2020

Recent studies from Harvard University confirm that the United Sates needs to significantly increase testing before opening the states, tripling the average of 145,000 tests per day to somewhere between 500,000 to 700,000 tests per day.

Despite these findings, governors in three Southern States plan to open beaches and small retail shops, including beauty salons and tattoo parlors, so they can "slingshot" around neighboring states that remain closed. Task force members and mayors in Georgia have voiced great opposition to this unilateral plan and complain that no one in the public health community was consulted.

It is sad to note that the death rate from the virus is still higher among African Americans, who account for 27% of all US deaths—two times higher than their share of the US population. No one knows the exact reason, but poverty and lack of health care are suspected.

The price of oil futures dropped to minus $40 per barrel, the largest one day drop in history which indicates there is more oil in the system than can be stored now that demand has suddenly fallen. In addition, dismal quarterly earnings—another leading indicator of economic health—sent the stock market down another 650 points today, with a total drop of 30% since mid-February.

APRIL 21, 2020

It has been sixteen days since the Swedish experiment to build herd immunity was reported in this journal. Deaths have increased to 1,765 today from 374 on April 4. The death rate is ten times that of their Nordic neighbors and it appears the experiment is doomed to failure but of course, only time will tell.

Tony Spell, the Louisiana pastor who bused thousands of people to his church services in March and April was arrested for using one of those buses to assault a lone protester who was standing on the sidewalk holding a sign that read "Close this church!" Later that afternoon, his supporters gathered wearing their Sunday best and bailed the pastor out of jail. Pastor Spell commented that he cannot "lay hands" on his parishioners if they are not in church, so he will not close.

Hydroxychloroquine is now considered a miracle cure by the president and his media supporters even though there are no studies to confirm the miracles, and many warnings about fatal side effects. "A beautiful drug," President Trump said several times during his recent White House briefings, which started a run on a medicine that patients with autoimmune disease desperately need and can no longer find.

However, studies released from three countries and the Veterans Administration indicate hydroxychloroquine does not help COVID patients, and there appears to be a ten percent higher death rate from the treatment. The drums for this drug have suddenly grown silent on Fox News but they still beat loudly in Brazil.

April 23, 2020

Unemployment figures for the past week were released with an additional 4.4 million Americans filing for unemployment which brings the total to 26 million new claims in four weeks. These people are mostly blue-collar—those who work for hourly wages to make goods and serve people; they have no savings and few options. There are lines of cars several miles long waiting for free food outside food banks in major American cities. Some people arrive just after midnight and sleep in their cars. This is what economic depression looks like in the new century.

On the flip side, workers at meatpacking plants in the South and Midwest—processing beef, pork and chicken—have high infection rates, but the plants are still open. Some reporters speculate that the governors of these Southern states do not want to pay unemployment claims. Georgia will open hair salons, tattoo parlors and gyms tomorrow. The state legislature, however, will conduct the peoples' business via Zoom until June.

We now know that more than one hundred Fortune 500 companies listed on the stock exchange—those with cozy banking relationships and good lobbyists—received billions of dollars meant for small businesses. The Personal Protection Program (PPP) quickly ran out of money while the "mom and pop" owners desperately tried and failed to reach their local bankers. You might wonder why the president fired the inspector general tasked with overseeing the two-trillion-dollar stimulus bill...or maybe you don't. There is no vision and no oversight, and the American dream is unraveling due to incompetence and greed...which makes our democracy ripe for autocracy.

April 24, 2020

The White House daily pandemic briefings were originally designed to bring information to the public from health professionals who sit on the White House Coronavirus Task Force. Vice President Pence ran the daily briefings until President Trump realized they were a low-cost opportunity for unlimited self-promotion. The VP was told to stand in the back while the president called on medical professionals and journalists, displaying a vast ignorance of science and facts. One afternoon he asked Mr. Pillow, a big donor, to lead the nation in prayer from the podium. Someone, please, loan our president a copy of the Constitution.

The briefings ballooned to two-hour presidential stream-of-consciousness events, with fewer and fewer health professionals standing quietly beside the king of magical thinking: the president of the United States.

This journal was not designed to be political, but politics have devolved our national pandemic response into a world-class disaster. On February 24, the president told the nation the virus was under control, and today—two months later—there are a million infected by official counts and an estimated ten million who were never counted due to the lack of federal testing. And still, he congratulates himself on national television every afternoon.

It seems President Trump finally went too far during the briefing yesterday. Alone at the podium, he asked the only medical professional seated nearby whether her team was looking into the benefits of sunlight as a cure. And then he asked if they were looking into how effective injecting or ingesting antibacterial cleaning agents might be, since they kill the virus on surfaces so quickly and might help the lungs. That night there were a hundred calls to the Maryland poison control center after people started drinking bleach.

The briefing today was less than twenty minutes with no questions from the press allowed because his aides finally convinced the president that these daily briefings could harm his re-election chances.

The Denver Metro Emergency Food Network has delivered 85,000 meals in six weeks.

APRIL 25, 2020

When polled, nearly seventy percent of Americans want the stay-at-home orders to continue until no longer necessary, but this is a difficult calculus since so much is unknown about the virus: How many known infections? How many are unknown? Can a recovered person be re-infected? What is the real death rate? How long before reliable antibody tests will be available? How far can the virus spread without masks? How far does it spread with masks? Will there be a second wave before a vaccine? Will there be a vaccine?

Most states (and countries) are considering these questions and trying to develop a rationale for opening businesses in May. Most health professionals have said it is too soon and most people seem to agree that without COVID safety measures they will be staying home. In states that never closed there are still no recommended protocols and no federal guidelines, just a chart with goals that have yet to be reached.

Japan is experiencing the consequences of not shutting down or adequately testing, much like the US. They are currently administering around 300 tests per day and just recently issued a stay-at-home order that the Japanese people are choosing to ignore. Their health care system is on the verge of collapse.

APRIL 26, 2020

Spring has finally arrived. Snow from the storm three weeks ago has melted, the trees are budding, the birds are active—especially the ruffed grouse drumming for mates—and the streams are running full and milky. The air is clear, and the night sky reveals a dense arc of stars that mark the far edge of the Milky Way.

All around the world people marvel at the clear air and night sky, especially where pollution has obscured the view for decades. In just two months, people have experienced the best air quality of the past twenty-five years: Los Angeles has the lowest pollution of any major city on earth; New Delhi has seen a 60% drop in pollution over this time last year; the mountains surrounding Beijing are suddenly visible for the first time in decades.

These environmental benefits may be fleeting, but they provide a clear reminder of the industrial harm we have inflicted upon the earth during the past century. Without human activity, the world cleans up nicely.

The pause in activity has also caused the collapse of the oil market, and the industry is beginning to shut down. Last week crude producers had to pay $50 a barrel to unload excess supply into tankers anchored offshore; dozens dot the water beyond the California coast. There are fifty million barrels going into storage every week, forty percent of wells have been shuttered, and refinery production is down by a third. Small producers and refineries may never recover.

This week the oil market opened at $16 a barrel, which is still more than the cost of production. A recent cartoon showed a man filling his gas tank and asking the station attendant, "So, what do you owe me?" I can't remember the last time I filled up.

The irony is that politicians denied climate science because it looked bad for the oil producers who funded their campaigns. Now it appears that vaccine science is the only way to restore the oil market.

APRIL 27, 2020

There were no virus briefings from the White House over the weekend. After canceling Monday's press briefing, a last-minute conference was called to announce "new" plans to address the testing needs of the nation. The president congratulated his task force on a great job and reported they had just surveyed all fifty governors to see what they needed to ramp-up testing. Of course, there was no offer of funding or oversight. They simply rebranded incompetence to sell as success.

Now that we have been living with this pandemic for two months, it is still stunning to realize how much we don't know...like how many people are dying from the virus. A recent investigation into additional US deaths in March discovered 15,000 more deaths than previously reported. Without testing, only death rates paint the true picture.

The tests we do have tell us very little. There are too many false negatives, and the positives require a buildup of virus; asymptomatic people could be spreading the infection but if they test too early, they will never know.

Michael Osterholm—an epidemiologist from University of Minnesota—summed up his analysis of testing with this chilling statement: "Testing won't get better until the pandemic gets worse."

We are almost through the first wave, and what we have learned might help with the second wave. Now that fourteen states have lifted some or all restrictions, the germs of that second wave are spreading now.

I am reminded of people being chemically treated for serious mental illness. They take medicine until they feel better and then stop because "they don't need it anymore."

And so goes our virus cycle: irrational people will not follow health advice to combat threats they cannot see.

APRIL 28, 2020

There is one fact about the spread of the virus we can believe because we see it: those living or working in small spaces without protection have the highest infection rate, a simple fact supported by common sense.

Who does this include? These forgotten souls who have been mentioned previously but are finally being counted: residents of nursing homes where nearly half the deaths in some states have occurred; inmates housed in overcrowded prisons with 80% infection rates; veterans by the thousands who are sick and dying in underfunded VA facilities.

The list also includes people with essential jobs that require shoulder-to-shoulder contact in meatpacking plants—home to 500,000 of our lowest-paid workers. Infection and absenteeism have closed some plants, but owners have warned that new safety measures could be a threat to the food supply. In a twist of logic, the CDC agreed to loosened safety regulations at the plants, replacing their usual stern warnings with suggestions and guidelines to use "only when feasible."

Trump then signed his second emergency production order requiring the plants to stay open although there are more than 3,000 sick and many hundreds dead already. He cites "liability issues" as his reason for the order, which means the owners are protected but the workers are not. And when the states open back up, those who do not return to work are no longer eligible for unemployment benefits.

The actions of our political and economic leaders highlight those who are expendable: The elderly, the sick, the lowest-wage earners and, of course, those who fought for our freedom during the past fifty years.

The world has reached a milestone today: three million (known) cases worldwide with a third of those cases—one million—right here in the richest country in the world.

APRIL 29, 2020

On February 25, The US announced an international trial of Gilead's antiviral drug called Remdesivir—developed in response to SARS and MERS—to treat COVID. Today the initial results were reported by Dr. Fauci in a White House press briefing. There were 1,009 participants in a blind study, and although not statistically significant due to the low sample size, researchers saw some improvement in duration of illness and mortality rate. Remdesivir will become a new treatment and there are already one million doses ready for hospital use. Investors obviously took a gamble.

The results of this drug trial were not scientifically conclusive and have not been replicated, leading some experts to suggest caution. In fact, another study in China showed no significant improvement. But hope springs eternal (with profits gushing upward) and the world really does need some good news for a change.

Also in the upbeat news department, the Denver Metro Emergency Food Network (DMEFN) reached a milestone of 100,000 meals delivered in the past forty-two days and earned more well-deserved publicity in the local news.

With expanded capacity using additional facilities, DMEFN hopes to reach 250,000 meals delivered by mid-June, another challenging goal. Rachel and Kevin volunteer every Sunday, standing six feet apart while chopping and assembling and packing up dinner boxes, talking through masks. Those of us who watch from a distance just send money. Fundraising is going well, and DMEFN has enough money (and goodwill) to deliver meals for another ten weeks.

APRIL 30, 2020

	CASES	DEATHS
WORLD:	3,358,157	237,091
US:	1,095,623	63,865

The US released unemployment figures for the past week: 3.8 million people successfully applied despite an overloaded system, bringing the unemployment insurance claims to over 30 million in six weeks. If you add the unemployment insurance claims prior to COVID, the total for the US is currently 36 million—the highest rate since the 1934 depression—meaning 22% of the American workforce is now receiving unemployment compensation.

In addition, there are between 9 and 14 million unemployed who either did not apply, tried and did not get through, or are still trying but have not succeeded, which indicates the unemployment rate will continue to climb beyond the current unprecedented number.

Every week there are comparisons between our current economic disaster and the Great Depression triggered by the stock market crash of 1929. Historic black-and-white photos of men in long lines, three or four abreast waiting for a meal at the soup kitchen, are juxtaposed with videos of drivers in mile-long lines waiting for boxes of goods to be placed in the trunk. Most of the people interviewed while waiting confide they have never been in such a position, but with no jobs there is no option: they must feed their families.

And this is just the beginning. Forbes estimates that some cities will see a 40% workforce reduction in the coming weeks, due to a dependence on high-risk industries like oil and energy or entertainment, including Las Vegas and Atlantic City, and Kahului, Hawaii, a state almost entirely dependent on tourism.

The Denver Metro Emergency Food Network delivered 15,000 meals this week.

MAY 3, 2020

Once again, it just feels wrong to watch a mob of men with AR-15 rifles invade the Michigan State House to protest mitigation measures designed to combat high infection rates and deaths in the state—measures that were recommended by the White House just a few days before President Trump decided to praise armed protesters instead.

Although politicizing the pandemic is not surprising in an election year, these people are putting themselves, their families, their communities, and the country at risk to protest lockdowns. They are spitting mad at those protecting the common good, and use props to threaten minorities including confederate flags, nooses, and swastikas.

Apparently, refusing to wear a mask or stand six feet apart is considered a mark of independence and strapping a rifle or gun to your body shows how serious you are. President Trump's base wants liberty without responsibility and the president wants power without consequences. They deserve each other.

But we the people deserve more than vanity and temper tantrums; we need real leadership to save the nation. This president was unfit from day one, but our laws allow corporations to buy and sell leaders as if they were stock options. Will we survive?

This virus is unconcerned with political parties or politicians, profit margins or markets, and is just getting started. This is the scene in the disaster movie when real danger emerges, and the camera focuses on the hero. “Better buckle up!” she says.

MAY 4, 2020

Sweden’s experiment in herd immunity continues. The country is still not in lock-down, has limited social distancing rules, and masks are not required or recommended. The health minister leading this experiment commented that they are not surprised by the high infections, but they are surprised by the number of deaths which have increased to 2,854 from 374 in the past thirty days.

Death is a high price for herd immunity—if immunity even exists without vaccines or extensive illness which is yet to be determined. Sweden’s death rate is 283 per million, the US rate is 218 per million and Sweden’s neighbors, Finland and Norway, have a death rate of 43 per million and 40 per million respectively. The news from Sweden is difficult to fathom, with so many young adults in the cafe and shops—shoulder to shoulder—while their elders fall like flies; most of the deaths have occurred in nursing homes.

Unthinking people comment that this pandemic is nature’s way of thinning the herd, of limiting the number of elderly, obese, diabetic and heart challenged patients in the world. Such tone-deaf rationales for letting people die have been rejected by the majority who love their mothers and fathers, sisters and brothers, and willingly stay home to protect them.

May 5, 2020

New York State has the highest death rate of any other state, county, city or neighborhood by 1000%. The US death rate for all states combined is 218, while in New York the rate is 1,285, followed by New Jersey at 934, Connecticut at 735, and Massachusetts at 617 per million.

Indications are that population density is a factor as well as health care accessibility, but even Manhattan with 27,000 people per square mile is not the most highly populated city in the world. If density were the only consideration, NY state would be in the middle of the death pack instead of leading it. The more likely cause is seriously inadequate health care for the poor and elderly and very early virus transmission.

Some believe the virus was running rampant in New York city a month or two before the first cases were diagnosed, indicating an initial spread over the 2019 Christmas holiday. With so many uninsured—and the distinction between flu and COVID not apparent—the early cases were not diagnosed; most people do not seek medical care for the flu and besides, there was no early test for COVID.

And then the wave hit, and the hospitals were overrun. People died in the hallways and their bodies were stored in refrigerator trucks that sometimes broke down. The hospital tents in Central Park are still unused, but this is just the first wave. The good news is that those states with early lockdowns have the fewest infections—including Oregon—but infection slowly moves west despite what we do.

Nearly forty-two states are now developing plans to open for business over the next month. Some of these states are at the beginning of the curve and will see COVID spikes followed by death over the next thirty days. Apparently, this risk is acceptable to those who see economic destruction as the greater of two evils, including President Trump who plans to phase out the Coronavirus Task Force. "Let's open this country back up!"

He needs a good economy for re-election since magical thinking only goes so far. Like Sweden, he has decided to let bodies fall where they will.

MAY 6, 2020

A trip to the grocery store in Wallowa County is an experience in extremes. On one side of town there is a Safeway store—part of a large supermarket chain—where safety protocols from headquarters have been implemented. Two weeks ago, I decided to shop during "senior hours" and showed up at 7 am along with a horde of other seniors.

Everyone was wearing masks and following the directional arrows on the floor…everyone except me who obviously needed special instruction. I wondered why people were staring at me and then felt like an idiot when I figured out the "no opposing traffic" rule. Grocery shopping is difficult during a pandemic.

Today I tried the locally owned store on the other side of town and discovered that not one in ten people was wearing a mask—not even the stockers or checkers. I felt like a leper in my surgical mask and mentioned to one young man stocking shelves, "I am wearing this for you!" He just rolled his eyes.

It is true that we only have one case, now recovered, and this conservative town religiously follows Fox News where some talking heads are saying that mitigation efforts are unnecessary, that the liberal media is making a big deal out of nothing. Even here, among neighbors, there is a partisan divide.

Our governor is negotiating with leaders in rural Oregon, and it looks like some restrictions will be lifted mid-month. The local community will welcome that, initially. But the danger for this resort town is that when the state opens for business, travelers will bring the virus here. We wonder if there is any viable alternative besides letting our neighbors go bankrupt, and quickly realize the only alternative is a vaccine.

MAY 7, 2020

The unemployment figures released today report another 3.2 million claims, for a total of nearly 40 million, which is a rate of 14.7%, the highest unemployment since the Great Depression (which was 15.9% in 1931).

Not wearing a mask has become an expression of "liberty" for the anti-government fringe, which led to the shaming and shooting of a store clerk in Flint, Michigan, who tried to enforce the mask rule at the Family Dollar store. We can expect more violence due to President Trump's recent tweet to "LIBERATE" the states.

The plan to open the states will not be tempered by social distancing, fear of infection rates, testing, or contract tracing. People need to go back to work and start spending money to stimulate the economy—an economy that threatens to create another one-term president—so caution is thrown to the wind.

But people are not fooled. A recent survey reported that 64% want the states to stay closed until it is safe to reopen. And still, the partisan divide is apparent: 92% of Democrats and 35% of Republicans want safety first. We are decidedly not all in this together.

MAY 8, 2020

Although the United States represents just five percent of the world's population, we have 33% of the COVID infections and our death rate is 232 per million compared to 34 per million in the rest of the world.

For decades, we have been told that for-profit health care means we are buying the best care in the world. Even so, we cannot keep up with a microscopic virus because we lack testing, protective gear, and contact tracing, which are common tools in a pandemic. More than a million non-crisis health care providers have lost jobs during the pandemic because ICU beds are in high demand and for-profit surgeries are not.

We are witnessing a cascade of failure from the top down, starting with a narcissistic leader representing vulture capitalism, an avalanche of inequality, an impoverished educational system, and the inability of our institutions to put the welfare of people ahead of profits. When we add a pandemic, the whole house of cards comes tumbling down. America is indeed exceptional in the world: To have so much wealth and still slide towards failure requires a staggering amount of greed.

The Denver Metro Emergency Food Network delivered 12,000 free meals to the jobless and hungry in Denver this week.

MAY 9, 2020

It is no surprise that the president's supporters do not follow the recommendations for social distancing and wearing masks, the only tools we have to fight the pandemic. President Trump also refuses masks, saying it is not "seemly" for someone who interacts with kings and queens to wear a face covering. Really.

Even when visiting a mask manufacturing plant, he did not wear a mask—only goggles for some unknown reason. In addition, the vice president did not wear a mask at the Mayo Clinic while visiting patients, which is required. In fact, no members of the president's cabinet, his task force, or his staff were allowed to wear masks in the White House…until now.

Two members of the president's staff have tested positive for COVID, including the valet who serves his meals and the spokeswoman for the vice president, a woman who met with reporters in close quarters without a mask the day before she tested positive—even though all the reporters were wearing masks. Three members of the virus task force are in quarantine.

Forty-eight states will be opening in phases within the week, and again there are some who claim their rights are being violated when they're asked to wear masks. Eleven men armed with assault rifles and a rocket launcher walked into a North Carolina Subway shop and announced it was their "God given right" to carry weapons and eat sandwiches without masks, although some wore bandanas like wild west bandits.

You must be stunningly insecure—and willfully ignorant—to need an assault rifle to buy a sandwich at Subway.

MAY 10, 2020

As usual I planted flowers on Mother's Day, a long tradition. Our bubble-mates (Don, his wife, Linda, and Marcy) came over to sit outside in lawn chairs and enjoy the beautiful day. We sat six feet apart throughout the afternoon, but it was too hot to eat in the yard, so we moved to the deck where we sat three feet apart…almost. Marcy will reopen her facial business this summer and then we will reconsider how much risk to take.

Wallowa county will open next weekend, and people are excited to get a haircut as soon as they can. I am worried that our "no virus" county will experience our first wave in a few weeks so I ordered a set of hairdressing tools and will try my hand at haircuts on the deck.

As more information is compiled about the symptoms of COVID, the prospect of contracting the virus is increasingly frightening. There can be severe complications involving the brain, organs, respiratory system, bones, muscles and other mysterious immune responses that have recently killed three young children in New York and sickened dozens more. There is no set of symptoms common to all and the recovery can take weeks and even months. The long haulers—those who have yet to heal—might suffer the rest of their lives.

The R0 (rate of infection) can range from one or less in a contained community to three or four if running rampant, which means one person can infect four, and they can infect sixteen, and they can infect sixty-four in just three degrees of contact. Our quarantine will continue.

MAY 11, 2020

It is strange to see photographs and videos of the Western world's greatest cities completely devoid of people in the streets, or museums, or restaurants, or historic places—including the Vatican where the Pope delivers mass to a completely empty St. Peter's Square.

There are reports of goats roaming the streets of Rome and pumas wandering in Santiago, jellyfish and rare seabirds swimming the canals in Venice and monkeys enjoying lunch in the middle of an empty marketplace in New Delhi.

There are herds of sheep in Istanbul and deer in London and rabbits hopping around Christchurch. Gaggles of geese, solitary peacocks, and wandering ducks are filling the void left by civilization in other major cities. It has been a mere two months since humans barricaded themselves behind doors, but sixty days is apparently long enough for the rest of the animal kingdom to feel safe in our deserted streets.

In the US, there are no final decisions regarding if, when, or how colleges will open campus this fall, or when major sports franchises including football and baseball will begin their seasons. Broadway will not open until September and there is no one offering a music concert anywhere in the nation…or anywhere in the world.

For two months the world has been in lockdown. The virus travelled so fast that no one was prepared, and now more than four million are infected and 280,000 (officially counted) are dead. It is nearly impossible to wrap your head around it.

MAY 12, 2020

Most public health professionals would agree that infections and deaths are underreported, especially in countries with authoritarian or repressive governments—including Russia, Pakistan, Saudi Arabia, India, Brazil, Turkey and China—where it is common to see a high number of infections and a low number of deaths reported.

But some countries have been successful in controlling the epidemic and report high testing rates and numbers of deaths per million in the single-digit range, an ideal situation. South Korea is an example, where there are currently 260 deaths in a country one-sixth the size of the US (or 55 million versus our 330 million). If their deaths were multiplied by a factor of six to compare (apples-to-apples) with the US, they would have around 1,560 deaths to our 83,000 to date.

It is obvious we are doing something wrong in this country and will see our failure in concrete terms as deaths rise over the next few months. Maybe we will learn that a deadly virus cannot be controlled by magical thinking.

MAY 14, 2020

Unemployment figures for the past week were released this morning. Another 2.9 million souls were successfully added to the rolls, bringing the total claims for two months to 36.5 million, still the highest two-month total ever recorded. Nearly half the low-wage workers in the US have lost their jobs including 40% of those households making under $40k.

We are grateful that all the young adults in our family are still employed. Rachel celebrated her 31st birthday with Kevin and Michael in Denver last night. They will soon become roommates since Rachel and Kevin are moving into the parental suite in Michael's home to save money starting in June.

As most of the states begin to open with no national plan, the model that predicts the death rate in the US has been adjusted upward: 147,000 deaths are expected before August 1.

Just a week after Trump's executive order keeping meatpacking plants open, infection rates in those counties increased by 40%. All fifteen counties with the highest COVID infections in the US are home to a meatpacking plant or a prison. Once again, we see that exposure in high-density situations—with people working or living closely together—can rapidly spread the virus.

In Wisconsin, the State Supreme Court struck down the governor's stay-at-home order. This was the same court that forced citizens to vote in-person recently, causing dozens of new infections. A few bars immediately opened, and we saw photos of people sitting shoulder-to-shoulder enjoying their "freedom."

In Michigan, the Republican legislature closed the Capitol to protect themselves from their own supporters who announced plans for another armed protest.

Wallowa County businesses will open tomorrow, and we plan to shop from a distance—to order by phone and pick up at the curb. Michael opened one of his coffee shops in Denver for take-out coffee and pastry orders; not sure this is a sustainable model for him, but it must feel good to try.

May 15, 2020

	Cases	Deaths	Deaths per million
World:	4,621,414	308,154	40
US:	1,484,285	85,507	270

Because we are retired and live on twenty acres of forest at the edge of the Oregon wilderness, our daily lives have not really changed. We read the news over two cups of coffee every morning, exercise several times a week, read or write or cook or sauna during the middle of the day, and watch a movie at night. Today we wandered around the property looking for morel mushrooms, like we do every May. We see my brother and his wife once a week because we know they also isolate, and we make occasional trips to the grocery store.

But we know that the urban/rural divide creates distinct pandemic experiences, as does the difference in risk between young and old and whether a person is liberal or conservative, white collar or blue, white skin or brown or black, middle class or poor, working or retired, with children or without. The term "global pandemic" means everyone is affected in some unique way.

But due to the dynamics of this election year, political affiliation is a direct indication of how serious a person regards the COVID risk. The pandemic has become a political football, but history shows this is no exception.

The 1918 pandemic—called the Spanish flu—occurred during WW1 and was downplayed to keep attention focused on the war effort. Workers who were spending their days loading ambulances or digging graves could only shake their heads in wonder when leaders ignored the growing pandemic; they wondered why the sick and the dead were never mentioned on nightly radio broadcast; why there were treason laws against reporting "flu" deaths.

We shake our heads a hundred years later when we hear President Trump make the most absurd statements to convince the American people they can return to work and save the economy (and his re-election chances.) Here are a few of the highlights:

"If we didn't do any testing, there wouldn't be so many cases."

"We really don't need a vaccine since the virus will go away on its own."

"Shutdowns are deadly because people can't leave their house."

"Who knows? It could be that testing is overrated."

The public health community does know—or did before Trump became president. The CDC was the gold standard for the entire world in disease response but now the agency's public health leadership has been sidelined by a president and his political appointees who do not embrace facts or science. Instead of leading the world, CDC scientists stand behind an ignorant showman and try to mitigate the damage; they risk their careers to tell the truth, which is still difficult since they have not been allowed to hold even one press briefing since March.

Yesterday the director of the CDC warned that there will be over 100,000 deaths in two weeks and that is a conservative estimate. In my view, the presidential election on November 3 is literally a matter of life and death.

In the good news category, Denver Metro Emergency Food Network has delivered 150,000 meals since March 18.

MAY 16TH, 2020

If we have "only" 100,000 cases by June 1, that will signal a slowdown, but this is unlikely since the consequences of a "liberated" public will be self-evident in two weeks.

Last night all three cable news stations broadcast the program "Graduate Together," an uplifting hour of art and music and testimonials by graduating seniors with an address by our former president, Barack Obama, a man of wisdom and grace who led the nation for eight years—the anti-thesis of our current president. It was a nostalgic and hopeful program and reminded us of the potential "we the people" can bring to the table.

This virtual graduation celebration is one of hundreds throughout the nation, a creative response to the shutdown of schools and the spring activities students look forward to, especially seniors at the end of their public education. It is a milestone that deserves recognition.

Enterprise high school will celebrate with a parade of decorated vehicles, one per family; they will drive down main street and then congregate on the football field for awards and speeches, masks required.

MAY 17, 2020

It seems that people in Wallowa County—and around the country—have confused the word "open" with "over" and have stopped wearing masks and practicing social distancing. In some states, aggressive protesters are harassing masked reporters covering the news; they hold signs about fake news and a hoax virus and scream into the faces of those trying to do their job. It looks like news reporting from a war zone.

On the other hand, the newly named, Multi-symptom Inflammatory Syndrome that is attacking children with serious illness leads parents to wonder if it will ever be safe to send kids back to school. The sick children were exposed several weeks earlier and had symptoms that did not seem to fit COVID at first, but then they developed rashes and fevers and heart weakness and breathing difficulties, and additional testing confirmed the virus was killing them.

Much of the current testing has produced a significant number of false negatives, meaning first tests cannot confirm COVID due to a low viral load. Initially, these patients were sent home but health experts have since learned that if they appear to have the virus and test negative, they should be retested.

The global scientific community is frantically working to understand transmission, expression of symptoms, development of treatment options, vaccines, antibody tests, the probability of future waves, and the likelihood of a mutation. In science, we find hope for humanity.

MAY 18, 2020

A group of Eastern Oregon pastors and lawyers—advocating for their God-given right to assemble—sued the governor of Oregon for issuing orders that limit church services. A judge in Baker County decided in their favor and declared that the governor's emergency orders were null and void for the entire state.

The Oregon Supreme Court disagreed with the judge and put a hold on the decision, pending review. The lawsuit does not represent the will of the people. In a recent poll, 80% of Oregonians said they would prefer to stay home until state public health officers determine it is safe to resume daily activities.

In California, a pastor opened his church for Mother's Day services against stay-at-home orders and on Monday a woman in attendance tested positive for the virus. Two hundred people were exposed and the pastor was infected.

There is news of rising rates of infection in nearly all the southern states that reopened against the advice of public health officials.

In Colorado, Michael had very little takeout business at his newly re-opened coffee shop, clearing just $75 last week.

MAY 20, 2020

A super-cyclone—the second largest in recorded history—is churning its way towards India and Bangladesh, forcing the evacuation of 2.5 million people into shelters that were not designed for social distancing. Many are afraid to leave their homes and must choose between the risk of drowning or the risk of catching a deadly virus.

After two years of heavy rain, the worst desert locust plague in seventy years is raging from East Africa to the Middle East, destroying crops and threatening famine for millions of people already battling COVID. According to a recent UN briefing, a swarm of 200 billion locusts—eating its weight in food each day—can consume as much as 84 million hungry people. Estimates are that the swarm will grow five hundred times its current size by June and invade thirty countries unless something is done.

Two dams in Michigan failed last night due to unusually heavy rain. A reported four to seven inches fell across the state, requiring the evacuation of 11,000 people amid floodwaters that could reach up to nine feet in the city of Midland by noon. The dams were cited for safety violations but never upgraded and could not withstand a once-in-500-years flood.

Conversely, wildfire risks are predicted to be sixty percent higher in California this season with fewer available firefighters and a dwindling budget. Drier weather and higher temperatures in Florida caused brush fires on several thousand acres last week amid predictions of an active fire season. The Forest Service is having serious discussions regarding how to keep COVID out of fire camp this summer.

Murder hornets are responsible for the death of several people each year in Japan and have recently arrived on the Pacific coast for the first time. Keith watched a single hornet kill a mouse with repeated attacks on a news video, which he said was "seriously frightening."

MAY 21, 2020

Numbers for new unemployment claims were released this morning indicating 2.4 million more workers lost their jobs. The numbers are still staggering and bring the total number of claims in the last nine weeks to 39 million—or 25% of the US workforce. For comparison, during the same week last year there were around 200,000 workers needing unemployment benefits—or 3.6% of the workforce.

COVID "super-spreaders" are people who do not realize they have the virus and then attend a large event at the apex of their virus bloom and infect others...especially in environments where they are shouting or singing. The only way to solve the problem of asymptomatic super-spreaders, is to reduce large gatherings, spend less time in crowds, and increase the use of masks in public.

In an interesting historical note, 150 years ago an Irish American cook known as "Typhoid Mary" infected fifty-three people with the disease before she was institutionalized for being an asymptomatic super-spreader. She spent twenty-five years under lock and key before the discovery of antibiotics. She was not allowed to knowingly spread the disease. Today, southern governors refuse to even require masks to stop a deadly virus, citing personal freedom.

The entire state of Alabama is the new national hotspot after ending stay-at-home orders to encourage commerce. In the capital city of Montgomery, there is just one ICU bed available due to a surge in COVID hospitalizations. Meanwhile, the governor announced that entertainment venues—theaters, bars, restaurants—can reopen this holiday weekend with no mask mandate. Can you imagine being an ICU nurse in Montgomery?

MAY 22, 2020

The release of a new study from Columbia University (reported in *The New York Times* May 2020) gave new meaning to the term "exponential" in relation to the COVID infection rate.

By measuring the rate of infections after stay-at-home orders were in place and then working backwards, researchers were able to quantify the consequences of the delay in closing the states.

It is estimated that 36,000 fewer people would have died from the virus if we had shut down the states just one week earlier—March 8 instead of March 15. If we had shut down on March 1, a staggering 54,000 fewer deaths would have occurred. Before shutdown, the infection rate doubled nearly every day; after shutdown, the infection curve flattened.

There is concern that the doubling effect will return once the shutdown has ended. But masks and distancing will help, and most people are not as eager for crowds as they were before the pandemic. Hopefully, new cultural norms for social interaction can mitigate a second wave.

The Denver Metro Emergency Food Network has delivered a total of 175,000 meals in nine weeks at a cost of nearly $70,000 per week. The expense makes it difficult for volunteers to continue beyond the resources at hand, so they plan a slow finish…and hope to serve meals through July.

MAY 23, 2020

Americans are on the move this holiday weekend. Every private campground in our county is filled with travelers from around the

Northwest. Restaurants and bars are open and there are few signs of social distancing or masks around town. The grocery stores are bursting with strangers who have found the most beautiful place in the state with no COVID…or so they think. Another case was just reported in Wallowa County, a local twenty-year-old recovering at home. His contacts will be traced to see if others have been exposed or infected.

All states are at risk from an increasingly mobile virus, especially this weekend. The Governor of Arkansas announced that spectator sports can resume even though the state had the highest one day rise in infections this week. Florida will host a youth baseball tournament with seventy teams and 1,500 family members attending. Alabama has opened summer camps, day care, state parks and schools even though they have no remaining hospital capacity. Keith reminds me that people are irrational most of the time.

Eighteen of the fifty states opening this holiday weekend have no mandatory mask requirement—including Oregon—even though public health officials consider this an essential tool to control infection. In the remaining thirty-two states the order is rarely enforced due to the risk of violence.

This weekend we remember the Americans who have died before us, including those who died in the past nine weeks from the deadliest virus in a hundred years.

MAY 25, 2020

It is understandable that people want to gather and socialize after the difficulty of the past ten weeks. Last night we watched a movie with characters crowded together eating pie and dancing and walking around Chicago. I felt a stab of grief and then a flash of fear, an irrational fear about what they might catch while sitting too closely together…and breathing. I find myself looking at the pre-pandemic world through a warped pandemic lens. Finding delight together is normal human behavior; fear of being together is not.

We have similar dilemmas here at home. Hannah wants to visit before she starts medical school in mid-June and wondered about bringing her roommates, a final outing before the end of an era. Portland is still in lockdown so there are no holiday crowds, but all three have boyfriends…and those boyfriends have jobs and other friends. Maybe they could sleep in the new trailer or the tent I suggest and without thinking Hannah says, "Really…the trailer?"

We are not post-pandemic yet, and letting down our guard might undo ten weeks of isolation. Besides, Hannah will feel responsible if we fall victim to the virus. Without tests or contact tracing or any cohesive national plan, all of us are engaged in blind decision making … and it is heartbreaking.

MAY 27, 2020

Now that the pandemic has been completely politicized as a re-election strategy, it is strangely accurate to look back three months and describe the progress of the pandemic as a "blue wave" first, with a "red wave" coming.

The large coastal cities—Seattle, New York, and Los Angeles—were hit with infected travelers returning from international destinations, who then spread COVID to crowded neighborhoods. The mayors and governors and voters in these cities and states are predominantly Democrat, and the "blue wave" began.

With heads buried in the sand, the federal government ignored the problem and required the governors of each state to handle the pandemic without the benefit of a national strategy. The blue governors saw the exponential infection rate and rushed to prepare as best they could, closing schools and businesses, searching for protective gear, begging for tests, and imploring the federal government for help. Unfortunately, there are credible reports that FEMA replenished the national stockpile by waiting for governors to find Personal Protection Equipment (PPE) and then swooping in to claim it.

Initially, some governors in red states also began preparing for COVID until President Trump tweeted support for the armed protestors in Democratic states and the message was received: Liberate the states, don't wear masks, consider public health warnings fake news—the pandemic will be over by Memorial Day.

Infection rates are now rising in Minnesota, Alabama, Mississippi, Arkansas, Florida, North Carolina and Nebraska, to name a few of the twenty states that have not flattened the curve. Republican states with large rural populations and diminished health care services are in trouble, especially those that did not expand Medicaid when they had the chance. The "red wave" is coming.

MAY 28, 2020

Another 2.1 million workers were added to the unemployment rolls last week, which brings the total to forty million filing for unemployment—25% of the American workforce since mid-March. Some are going back to work so the current unemployment figures may be lower, but it is difficult to sort out.

The stock market has gained a thousand points due to corporate bailouts and new hope. The death toll has reached a grim milestone: 100,000 dead in ten weeks, mostly the elderly in nursing homes and the minorities without adequate healthcare and the low-wage earners in meatpacking plants. Welcome to America's twilight zone.

In the beginning, the virus was mainly a risk to the elderly, given the high death rate in nursing homes around the world, but eventually we learned that this virus attacks weakness wherever it's found—any person with an underlying chronic disease, without adequate nutrition or healthcare, without protection in high-risk situations; any place where people live or work closely together, in churches and prisons and factories, and in multi-generational households.

The virus also highlights collateral weakness: the economic fear of a nation with severe inequality, and the emotional stress of people who can no longer hug loved ones, and the physical exhaustion of parents suddenly crowded together under the same roof, caring for children while working. The virus attacks our lives from all sides.

Tonight, Rachel and Kevin are moving in with Michael to save on expenses in advance of their wedding. There goes our wonderful "parental suite" in Denver.

MAY 29, 2020

To shift blame for the staggering numbers of infections and deaths from the COVID virus in the US, President Trump accuses China and the WHO for not being honest about the facts. His attacks are harming our already tenuous relationship with China, although some might have merit. He has decided to pull US support for the WHO due to a perceived "bias" in favor of China. The president picks a political fight in the middle of a pandemic—a global killer that requires all hands-on deck.

Our national response is waning. There are too few press briefings by the CDC, the Coronavirus Task Force is apparently winding down, and the Republican members of Congress and the Senate are refusing to wear masks in chambers, meeting rooms, or even crowded elevators. Apparently, the president's supporters feel compelled to show their loyalty by ignoring common sense.

Meanwhile, the emergency declaration by President Trump to open the meatpacking plants had the expected outcome at a Tyson pork-processing plant in Iowa: 22% of the 2,500 workers have now tested positive for the virus and the plant is shutting down. To date, 17,000 meat processing workers have tested positive for the virus and sixty-six have died. Most of these plants are in the Midwest where the infection rates are rising. Tyson cited a lack of testing as the reason so many workers were infected and still on the job.

MAY 30, 2020

	Cases	Deaths	Deaths/Million
World:	6,150,482	370,506	47.5
US:	1,816,820	105,557	319

Across the nation there is growing anger due to the murder of an unarmed Black man by four White police officers in Minneapolis on May 25. George Floyd was arrested and handcuffed after a 911 call about a $20 counterfeit bill, and a responding senior officer kneeled on his neck until he was dead. Several witnesses recorded video while others yelled for the officer to stop. "You are killing him!" they cried. The four White officers have been fired and one (so far) has been charged with third-degree murder.

There have been large protests in a dozen cities over the past four nights including Washington DC. The White House has gone dark and is in lockdown tonight, and President Trump briefly retreated to an underground bunker. He has inflamed the situation with a threatening tweet this morning: "When the looting starts, the shooting starts." A precinct building and a nearby restaurant in Minneapolis were burned to the ground Wednesday night.

The Boogaloo Bois, wearing Hawaiian shirts and carrying weapons, have infiltrated the protests and incited violence, just as they did during the lockdown protests in Democratic states. The goal of these anarchists—who have organized online—is to spark a civil war and any protest will do. They pose as members of an anti-fascist movement to confuse authorities.

It is important to note that White men armed with automatic rifles were allowed to occupy the Michigan State House without pushback by police, but unarmed Black protesters in Minnesota were greeted by tanks and troops in riot gear, state troops that were throwing tear gas cannisters and flash bang shells into peaceful protesters.

The Denver Metro Emergency Food Network has delivered 200,000 meals since March 18th. Their work has been recognized by Colorado Senator Bennett, PBS, Denver CBS, and several newspapers to date; there are several videos available on YouTube.

MAY 31, 2020

Say his name.

George Floyd was killed by four White police officers last week. Tonight, we mark the sixth night of protests and riots that have spread to thirty cities across the US, including Portland and Denver. An early curfew is being enforced in forty cities across twenty states.

Thousands of unarmed people are in the streets, standing together to protest police brutality, and there are hundreds of police and national guard troops facing them using tear gas, rubber bullets, flash bangs, batons, tanks and pepper spray to disperse the crowds. It looks like a military occupation.

Some police officers are aggressive, and this seems more like an "us versus them" battle, not the exercise of a solemn pledge to keep the peace during a legal protest. In a tweet, President Trump threatens to "unleash vicious dogs and ominous weapons" upon the protesters at the Capitol.

But some enforcement officers recognize a sea change: What the world witnessed on May 25 was a White policeman with his knee on the neck of an unarmed Black man for nine minutes and twenty-nine seconds, causing his death. Those who call this a lynching in broad daylight by a Minneapolis police officer are not exaggerating.

Although we have seen some rioting and anarchy—looting and the destruction of property with Molotov cocktails—most of the protesters are peaceful and appalled by the racism displayed against Black Americans in this country. People of every color are gathering despite danger from police using excessive force—or a possible COVID infection.

We know that ten percent of those infected are responsible for eighty percent of the spread—known as super spreaders—so if a few have the virus at these nationwide protests, hundreds could be infected. When you add the shouting and the shoving and the coughing from tear gas, the risks become exponential.

On another note, two NASA astronauts in a privately-owned rocket blasted into space this afternoon to rendezvous with the orbiting space station, the first manned flight from US soil in nine years… funded by a billionaire.

JUNE 1, 2020

Seven days of protest

My head is spinning, and it is hard to know where to start a description of events over the past 48 hours. I think Ryan O'Connor, city manager of St. Paul, said it best when he noted the triple threat to American cities: The biggest health crisis since the flu pandemic of 1918, the largest economic crisis since the Great Depression, and the greatest social unrest since the late 1960s…when my generation took to the streets to protest the Vietnam War—a war during which 58,000 Americans lost their lives (which is still only half the pandemic toll to date.) "Drugs, sex, and rock-n-roll" was the rallying cry of the young protestors who were desperate to throw off the yoke of a senseless war machine.

Our triple threat is now being illustrated with a symbolic math equation: 1918 (Spanish Flu) + 1929 (Depression) + 1968 (Civil Rights Movement) = 2020

Keith and I were driving home from La Grande and listening to reports of a large peaceful protest across from the White House in Lafayette Park when the announcer suddenly sounded alarmed. Apparently, hundreds of troops in riot gear and on horseback appeared and started attacking the crowd, pushing them back from the public space where they were legally assembled. Screams and blasts could be heard over the announcer's voice. "I don't understand why they are doing this," he said as everyone ran.

An hour later it became crystal clear. President Trump assembled the press for a Rose Garden speech and threatened to invoke the insurrection act of 1807—to deploy thousands and thousands of armed American troops against American protesters without consent from the governors.

Then Trump walked down the now empty street adjacent to the park, climbed the steps to a vandalized church, and held up a bible for the cameras. He did not ask for calm, he did not pray, and he did not notify the church that he was planning to visit. He used the church and the bible as a backdrop in his culture war against people of color, in his battle to make White people great again. He is at war with America.

The American system of government is teetering on the brink while the entire world watches in alarm at how quickly the nation is failing. President Trump adds fuel to every fire, seemingly energized by the chaos but devoid of the leadership skills needed to respond to a crisis. The world sees a wanna-be fascist dictator which they have seen many times before…but never in America.

Protesters realize their movement against police brutality is harmed by the anarchists who infiltrate peaceful protests and incite violence; organizers are screening participants more carefully. The public and police chiefs and state leaders around the nation are realizing that racism has infected the nation's police force and criminal justice system since the end of the Civil War, first through lynchings, and then Jim Crow laws, and now (really, always) through crushing economic and social inequality.

Police brutality is unfolding before our very eyes, as evidenced by the excessive force suffered by protesters in every state, and by reporters who have also been arrested without cause or shot with rubber bullets or sprayed with stinging tear gas on live TV. Police officers have also sustained injuries, unfortunately.

The murder of George Floyd tipped the nation into a watershed moment and the world is laser focused to see if America will sink or swim. The world understands: "As goes the part, so goes the whole."

JUNE 2, 2020

Eight days of protest

An Australian news team was filming the peaceful protest in Lafayette Park when it suddenly turned violent, and fully-armed troops forced people to run for their lives. The international reporters were attacked by military police and the video has gone viral around the world (like the pandemic). The Australian government has vowed to launch an investigation.

There have been protests at US embassies in a dozen countries, and foreign newspapers write, "Edge of an Abyss!" to describe what is happening here. Leaders from all over the world are condemning President Trump.

Today there were peaceful protests in 140 American cities and in every state including Mississippi, the last holdout. Hundreds of thousands of American citizens gathered and demanded that the US reform laws governing the police and the use of force that has allowed centuries of racial injustice.

Today, in a startling confirmation of excessive force, dozens of armored vehicles rolled down the streets of Washington DC, while troops fanned out around the Capitol and military police marched to the Lincoln Memorial to line the steps in descending rows just after a peaceful protest ended—a protest of all ages and colors who listened to speeches and prayers and repeated reminders to respect the curfew, which they did.

An iconic photo of military police surrounding Lincoln's statue—the president who ended slavery—to guard it from those who peacefully gathered to protest racial injustice will forever document one of the most serious threats to democracy this generation has witnessed.

The authoritarian measures promised and celebrated by this president have doubled the size of protests across the nation and led to outrage. And the fact that military troops attacked a peaceful protest so President Trump could stage a photo op has galvanized the world against him.

Is this a turning point? Will we reject authoritarian leadership, White supremacy, and vulture capitalism? Will we finally become a nation of all people, by all people, for all people?

Not without a fight, it seems.

JUNE 3, 2020

Nine days of protest

Today I submit a statement from General Jim Mattis, a highly decorated and well-respected military man with fifty years of service. He was the first Defense Secretary of the Trump administration but resigned in protest eighteen months later over the treatment of allies. He has not spoken or written a word about President Trump before this statement, which was published in *The Atlantic* today.

IN UNION THERE IS STRENGTH

General Jim Mattis (Retired)

June 3, 2020

I have watched this week's unfolding events, angry and appalled. The words "Equal Justice Under Law" are carved in the pediment of the United States Supreme Court. This is precisely what protesters are rightly demanding. It is a wholesome and unifying demand—one that all of us should be able to get behind. We must not be distracted by a small number of lawbreakers.

The protests are defined by tens of thousands of people of conscience who are insisting that we live up to our values—our values as people and our values as a nation.

When I joined the military, some 50 years ago, I swore an oath to support and defend the Constitution. Never did I dream that troops taking that same oath would be ordered under any circumstance to violate the Constitutional rights of their fellow citizens—much less to provide a bizarre photo op for the elected commander-in-chief, with military leadership standing alongside. We must reject any thinking of our cities as a "battle space" that our uniformed military is called upon to "dominate." At home, we should use our military only when requested to do so, on very rare occasions, by state governors. Militarizing our response, as we witnessed in Washington, D.C., sets up a conflict—a false conflict—between the military and civilian society. It erodes the moral ground that ensures a trusted bond between men and women in uniform and the society they are sworn to protect, and of which they themselves are a part. Keeping public order rests with civilian state and local leaders who best understand their communities and are answerable to them.

James Madison wrote in Federalist 14 that "America united with a handful of troops, or without a single soldier, exhibits a more forbidding posture to foreign ambition than America disunited, with a hundred thousand veterans ready for combat." We do not need to militarize our response to protests. We need to unite around a common purpose. And it starts by guaranteeing that all of us are equal before the law.

Instructions given by the military departments to our troops before the Normandy invasion reminded soldiers that "The Nazi slogan for destroying us...was 'Divide and Conquer.' Our American answer is 'In Union there is Strength.'" We must summon that unity to surmount this crisis—confident that we are better than our politics.

Donald Trump is the first president in my lifetime who does not try to unite the American people—does not even pretend to try. Instead, he tries to divide us. We are witnessing the consequences of three years of this deliberate effort. We are witnessing the consequences of three years without mature leadership. We can unite without him, drawing on the strengths inherent in our civil society. This will not be easy, as the past few days have shown, but we owe it to our fellow citizens; to past generations that bled to defend our promise; and to our children.

We can come through this trying time stronger, and with a renewed sense of purpose and respect for one another. The pandemic has shown us that it is not only our troops who are willing to offer the ultimate sacrifice for the safety of the community. Americans in hospitals, grocery stores, post offices, and elsewhere have put their lives on the line in order to serve their fellow citizens and their country. We know that we are better than the abuse of executive authority that we witnessed in Lafayette Square. We must reject and hold accountable those in office who would make a mockery of our Constitution. At the same time, we must remember Lincoln's "better angels," and listen to them, as we work to unite.

Only by adopting a new path—which means, in truth, returning to the original path of our founding ideals—will we again be a country admired and respected at home and abroad.

JUNE 4, 2002

Ten days of protest for racial justice

Another 1.9 million people applied for unemployment benefits last week, bringing the total to over forty-two million workers filing initial claims since late March.

This number does not include the almost two million who cannot work due to a positive COVID test, or those who care for the hundreds of thousands who are sick at home; this number does not include those who are undocumented, those who have given up looking for work or exhausted their benefits during the first wave.

Soon we must count the ones who have no daycare and can't return to work and those with no place to live due to foreclosure and those who have no transportation after their cars are impounded or failed to start. Someday we will understand that protestors not only march against racial injustice but against the economic injustice caused by extreme capitalism that has been highlighted during the pandemic. Someday the ranks of those protesting global inequality might swell into the millions, or maybe hundreds of millions before the quest for profit at-any-cost ends.

JUNE 5, 2020

There are racial injustice protesters by the tens of thousands in all twenty-five virus hotspots in the US and infection spikes in twenty states, so the US curve is going up again. But the federal government has ended all efforts to keep the nation informed. Dr. Fauci and the president have not spoken in nearly three weeks and there have been no public briefings or announcement regarding the rising curve or our inadequate response, and the testing czar is stepping down.

We are uplifted to see medical students and hospital employees line the sidewalks and cheer for protestors or simply kneel for nine minutes and twenty-nine seconds—the length of time the police officer held his knee on George Floyd's neck—to express solidarity with the national outrage over police brutality.

There are also global protests in various cities around the world with tens of thousands of people sending a message of support to America, protests that have evolved into a call for police reform in their own countries due to brutality towards minority populations.

"Power corrupts, and absolute power corrupts absolutely," Lord Acton wrote in 1887, highlighting a well-known human characteristic.

Civilization requires the imposition of a set of rules and then fair enforcement. We invest power in a system of laws and consequences and place our trust in those chosen to serve the public good according to those laws. We pay taxes to support a military presence to protect us from foreign threats, and a police force to protect us from domestic threats, including criminal behavior and natural disasters. Problems arise when the majority seeks to subject the minority to a secondary status using unfair laws and a jaded police force; problems arise when the law is used to institutionalize prejudice and maintain a hierarchy of privilege for those who make the laws.

Today we see President Trump appealing to those who support the hierarchy, inciting fear and attacking protesters for political purposes. He has referred to American citizens exercising their first amendment rights as thugs and terrorists; he has authorized thousands of unidentified troops to surround the capitol—a secret police force—erecting tall barricades around the White House and using tear gas and pepper spray and rubber bullets to intimidate peaceful protesters…and it works. Some police officers have betrayed their pledge to "protect and serve" and have promoted brutality against protestors, proving the point.

We understand there is police brutality in America; now we see there is endemic police brutality against Black Americans. Whether America can change is yet to be seen, but democracy surely depends on it.

JUNE 6, 2020

I would like to share a poem I stumbled across in the comment section of a NYT article. George Floyd cried out MAMA! just before he died under Derek Chauvin's knee.

There is an aspect to the George Floyd killing that made it intimately personal. It is hard to hate a man, but easy to hate a race. This poem speaks to George Floyd, the man, at his most vulnerable moment.

MAMA

I am a black mother,
And I heard you, George.
I watched the life drain from you,
And I saw my son's face.
Rage filled me at your suffering

and the indifference to your pain
and death.
Like a bear protecting her cubs
I wanted to strike, to tear, and to rend
But when I heard you cry for me,
All I could do was cry out for you
In return

I am a white mother,
And I heard you, George.
I saw that cop, and I saw my son's face
How he so casually betrayed you
How cruelly and inhumanely
He acted.
And I was ashamed and horrified.
I wanted to speak, to shout,
"Get off of him! Get off of him!"
But he didn't hear me, just as
You had not been heard,
When you cried out for your mama,
All I could do was cry for you
In return

I am the Earth mother,
And I heard you, George.
I felt your heart as it strove to beat,
Your lungs as they tried to fill.
I am mute witness to your suffering,
And the suffering of all of my children
Who've gone before you,
And I am here to receive you.
Lay down your body, George,
and rest.

Your work is done.
And I will hold you.

I am your mother, George.

—Nina Taylor
(from the NYT comment section)
Palm Harbor, FL
June 5, 2020

JUNE 7, 2020

Although Black Americans make up thirteen percent of the population, they have suffered twenty-three percent of the deaths from COVID, suffocating alone in an intensive care unit, terrified because they can't breathe, thinking about the loved ones they will soon leave behind.

"I can't breathe!" has become a rallying cry for two pandemics happening simultaneously in the Black community (three if you count economic devastation) and they knowingly risk one pandemic to fight the other: police brutality.

And it is not just COVID—that virulent microscopic exploiter of weakness—but all the diseases that strike down more Blacks per capita in this country. These Americans die of heart disease or diabetes, or kidney failure caused by the lack of healthcare and quality education…the legacy of institutionalized segregation, the hallmark of racism in America.

JUNE 8, 2020

New York City—the epicenter of the pandemic in the US—begins phase one reopening today. Although the NY curve has come down, the US curve has gone up in the past week due to higher rates in large states like Florida and Texas, states that reopened early and now have more than a thousand new cases a day.

During the Memorial Day holiday (two weeks ago) there was a dramatic shift away from stay-at-home orders and we are now seeing the results. The impact that hundreds of thousands of protesters might have on new cases will be clear in another two weeks.

But in twenty-two states the curve is now rising, including fourteen states with a fifty percent increase in the seven-day rolling average over the past five days. Hospitals in Arizona are nearing capacity, and the governor is now dusting off hospital emergency plans developed after re-opening early on May 15.

President Trump has tired of the health crisis and is now barricaded in the White House behind a ten-foot fence. Dr. Fauci is speaking up, however, reminding us that the past four months have brought devastation to the world and warning that the pandemic is far from over. The new death projection for the US is 145,000 dead by August 1—another 30,000 dead from COVID in seven weeks.

A new surge in Oregon is due to a cluster at a fishing plant, and another at an agriculture facility that infected dozens of workers. We worry that once these businesses close, people might decide to fuel up the motorhome and quarantine here. The Wallowa Lake state campground opens today and there is a steady stream of vehicles and visitors. There is another case of COVID in Wallowa County, another young adult recovering at home. No one is out of the woods yet.

JUNE 9, 2020

The protests are starting to have an effect. Several states have banned the use of chokeholds and neck-kneeling during arrests. Other states have changed secrecy laws to allow the release of abuse complaints against individual officers. Police unions are under fire for protecting the "bad" cops, and those who violate the rights of protesters are now being arrested. The public is wondering why civilian police forces need half a billion dollars of "surplus" military hardware offered by the federal government.

NASCAR and country music stars are throwing off the cloak of White supremacy—including Confederate flags and antebellum charm—and Hollywood is holding the industry accountable, calling for more diversity in films and awards going forward. The NFL has realized that taking a knee during the national anthem is a peaceful protest; owners and players have apologized for the seemingly racist reaction last year.

The two generals who walked with the president to Lafayette Square—after peaceful protesters were forcibly removed—have also apologized. Many high-ranking officers now say it was wrong for the "non-partisan" military to support such political actions.

However, the number of people still saying racist things out of habit is astounding, and there is little forgiveness when social media can easily record and distribute such offensive remarks; there have been quite a few sudden resignations.

But Trump continues to court his non-college-white-male base. He attended a roundtable with police in Dallas and neglected to invite the top three local law officers (three were Black and two were female.) He made statements praising the military police in Lafayette Square who cut through the protesters "like a knife through butter." President Trump never mentioned George Floyd in his visit with police, but his verbal assaults on citizens exercising their First Amendment rights are endless and anxiety-provoking.

Trump's most memorable speech regarding racism was after the Charlottesville White supremacy march in 2017 when he told us there were "very fine people on both sides," including the ones wearing hoods and holding torches, and the guy who ran down a female protester with his car, killing her.

Trump is planning a rally in Tulsa, Oklahoma next Friday, June 19. For the Black community, this day is celebrated as Juneteenth—a day set aside to honor emancipation of the slaves and to remember the 1921 massacre of Black Americans at Black Wall Street in Tulsa, the largest massacre of Blacks in our history. Is it just a coincidence that our racist president plans a rally in that town, on that day?

However, it appears the Black Lives Matter movement will not be stopped. There are still dozens of protests in cities around the world proving that Black lives do matter.

Perhaps—after suffering through this disastrous presidency—the ultimate result of our collective despair will be the uplifting of human character both here and abroad. We can dream; perhaps we *are* dreaming.

June 11, 2020

The virus marches on…actually, *through* the human population. My original goal was for a six-month journal—and today is the halfway mark—but it will likely be a year before we gain the upper hand on COVID. So, I will record events as long as the danger is with us… including from the threat of a dictatorship. This journal is for our children's children, and they deserve a full accounting.

In three months, we have gone from a total of 118,000 cases in the world to 7.5 million, and as some epidemiologists put it, "We are only in the second inning of a nine-inning game."

In the US, the next inning is likely to favor the virus since we benched the ace pitcher and scrambled the all-star infield and went to the refreshment counter instead of keeping our eye on the game. The virus is running the bases in twenty-two states, doubling the number of infections in just two weeks—from Memorial Day to the present.

Some say the rise in cases is due to increased testing, but the percentage of positive tests is rising and so is the score—virus 10, people 1. We get one point for closing down initially—saving the world from sixty million infections according to the referees—but we still have no real defense for the long game.

After a quick and confusing recovery, the Dow Jones lost 1862 points today due to the realization that we have a slow-moving first wave of infections after opening the states too soon. Last week another 1.5 million new claims for unemployment were filed, which also dampened the financial mood.

The statistics for Oregon released today show more than a double rise in infections—177 in 24 hours—including a cluster in La Grande due to a church that continued to hold services despite the order to close. The Oregon Health Authority is setting up a mobile testing site tomorrow since everyone who attended those church services is considered at risk for the virus. So far, there are five confirmed positive with two in the hospital which does not bode well for the church or the community. There is also another case here in Wallowa County.

JUNE 12, 2020

Last month the Oregon Supreme Court overruled a Baker County judge who wanted to end the Governor's emergency pandemic orders and open churches in Eastern Oregon. The court said there was no legal limit to the 28-day emergency stay-at-home order, ruling in favor of the governor.

Now, with an outbreak at the Lighthouse Church in La Grande, we can see what happens when churches remain open during a pandemic. Super spreader events often occur at gatherings where people sing and shout and dance around...like at political rallies and protests.

The White House claims 300,000 supporters have applied online for 19,000 tickets to the indoor Tulsa rally, signing a waiver to forgo legal action if they get the virus at the event. There is no cautionary message to those feeling ill, no announcement of specific social distancing guidelines, no recommendation that people wear masks. *Come at your own risk despite the risk* is the rallying cry from President Trump's campaign.

There are 20,000 new cases of virus confirmed in the US per day and rising. Tulsa saw a new peak in daily cases, along with the states of Florida, Texas, Alabama, Arkansas, North Carolina, South Carolina, and Oregon—hotspots beating their own daily records.

It appears that Oregon is seeing a rise in infections and the governor has put a pause on the reopening strategy...a "yellow light" for the next seven days to see where the infection rate is headed. We are still at the low end of the scale for deaths per million.

Hannah is on her way home without roommates, and thunderstorms are predicted for the next four days which means we remain indoors. It will be very awkward trying to social distance under the same roof, a dilemma many of my friends are facing. She starts medical school (initially online) next week and will be studying, but I was hoping the weather would allow for outside dining.

Everyone is making sacrifices, especially with the ones they love. Vacations, weddings, graduations, family reunions, sporting events, potlucks, concerts and other large gatherings have been canceled for the foreseeable future, but we are now permitted to gather with family members if we keep our distance...but no hugs. That will be weird.

The Denver Metro Emergency Food Network has delivered over 220,000 meals in the Denver area since March 18.

JUNE 13, 2020

The outbreak at Lighthouse church in La Grande turns out to be a catastrophe unfolding in real time. As public health director, Keith is informed of all new cases in Union County which includes the city of La Grande—one of the largest cities in eastern Oregon with 13,000 residents.

Two hundred members were tested for COVID at the mobile testing lab outside the church on Friday and 106 were positive. Another two hundred results are due tomorrow and then officials will inform the public that the infection rate has grown from five to 106 confirmed cases at the very least, and maybe a hundred more before the outbreak is under control.

Officials will then start testing everyone who was in contact with the initial 350; nearly all residents in this corner of rural Oregon will need to review where they went and with whom they spoke and if they wore a mask during the contact. There have been emergency meetings with state officials trying to determine the best way to proceed because the outbreak has already spread beyond the Lighthouse Pentecostal church. Apparently, the church continued to hold hands-on services, study groups, meetings, weddings and funerals despite the stay-at-home order, and then lied to public health and police officers who heard rumors and investigated.

All the fears about community spread and an overwhelmed hospital system are about to be realized close to home. Officials are counting ICU beds and ventilators in a hundred-mile radius, and we have yet to hear how the governor will respond.

Three counties in Eastern Oregon advanced to a Phase 2 opening on June 5th which permitted church activities if held outdoors by people wearing masks. Now it is likely our part of the state will need to phase back to increased isolation and the flow of summer travel to the area will cease. Due to the magical thinking of these self-centered believers, more neighbors could die, and more businesses might fail.

JUNE 14, 2020

Twenty days of protests for racial justice

Another Black man was killed by police outside a Wendy's in Atlanta last night, which was burned to the ground a few hours later by angry protesters. Rayshard Brooks, a father of three, was drunk and fell asleep at the wheel while waiting for his order at the drive-through window. The first officer was polite and told him to move his car and sleep in the parking lot, but a second officer forced him out of the car for a sobriety test, tried to taser him when he resisted being handcuffed, and then shot him twice in the back when he grabbed the taser, started to run and turned to fire.

Some call this use of force justified…but really? Why not take his keys and ID or license number and just let him sleep it off? Or let him run until he stumbles and arrest him then. Two shots in the back reeks of punishment not public safety. The officer was fired, the police chief resigned, and the mayor of Atlanta is "angry as hell."

Today is day twenty of the global protests in support of the Black Lives Matter movement. Some have been infiltrated by members of the far-right (and White) militia—not anti-fascists as President Trump claims—and their armed opposition to the racial justice movement again proves the point: the days of unchecked White privilege around the world are numbered; the movement to end institutional racism can no longer be stopped by violence.

Many writers and politicians and entertainment figures think this is a moment unparalleled in world history as the veil of racism and inequality—tolerated by majorities for so long—has been pulled back, exposing the rules and habits that torment minorities. Van Jones of CNN wrote an opinion piece titled, "Welcome to the Great Awakening," and expressed awe at the miracle of hope he now feels for his two Black sons. I challenge my own thoughts daily.

In local news, we are waiting for the press release announcing the large spike of cases in the nearby town of La Grande, and the steps necessary to deal with the outbreak, soon to be the largest in the state. Rumors have been flying around town and the anger towards the church is palpable. The only action possible is to identify those infected, treat the sick, and change minds about the threat of the virus even in rural Oregon communities. The pandemic is real.

JUNE 15, 2020

	Cases	Deaths	Deaths/Million
World:	8,108,667	438,596	43
US:	2,182,950	118,283	357

As diplomatic as the press releases have been about the outbreak at Lighthouse church, there are also videos of packed and boisterous church services circulating around the web and the story has been picked up by the news media including NBC and FOX outlets in Portland. The media reported ninety-nine new cases related to the church yesterday, for a new total of 205 in Union County with more to follow. The church is now closed, and their social media pages have been scrubbed.

A few anarchists on social media tried to pin blame for the surge on police brutality protests held last week, and claimed people were bussed in from all over the state, but this propaganda is distributed via far-right media networks and deposited into the mainstream.

Most people can see visual proof of dangerous gatherings inside the church as opposed to the images of peaceful protestors in masks standing quietly on the courthouse steps. Pictures of an inside wedding with two hundred guests have also been circulating, many of whom will likely test positive for COVID.

This local outbreak is a microcosm of the whole as evidenced by the increase of positive tests and hospitalizations in the red states that opened early, including Texas, Arkansas, Florida, Alabama, Mississippi, and Arizona.

In Arizona, restaurants were only allowed to open on May 15th, and then the bars and nightclubs saw a loophole and offered snacks to qualify. There were no other state requirements and soon nightclubs were packed with lines around the block, and people from nearby states flocked to Arizona and partied like it was 2019. Infections and hospitalizations have doubled to an all-time high while ICU availability in the state has fallen to 20%.

The governor of Arizona decided people should not be subject to blanket rules but should depend on their own good judgement… which is currently lacking in every corner of the country. The newest projections show a doubling of deaths by the end of September—over 200,000; without significant behavior change all bets are off.

As usual, we cannot look to the federal government to help us through the pandemic. Trump again suggested we stop testing altogether so there wouldn't be any more cases. He still plans to hold the

Tulsa rally for 20,000 supporters on Saturday despite the mayor and editorial boards in Tulsa pleading that he reconsider.

President Trump's re-election campaign reports that a million people have requested tickets, and some are already lining up outside the indoor stadium in downtown Tulsa. He is the hottest ticket in town…literally, infectious.

JUNE 16, 2020

Out of the 365 COVID tests conducted at the Lighthouse Union Pentecostal Church, 236 were positive which translates to a 66% positive infection rate. The average positivity rate nationwide is around 5%.

Oregon is now in the top five states for increasing infection rate due to the clusters in two seafood plants on the Oregon coast and the outbreak at the Pentecostal church. However, these clusters are not indicative of the rate in the entire state, thank goodness. Oregon is still in the bottom third of states for infection.

The most impressive increases are in Texas, Arizona, California, and Florida where the number of infected per day is doubling on a regular basis. Today there were 25,000 new infections in the US, and more than half were from those four states.

Vice President Pence—who leads the virus task force—published an op-ed in *The Washington Post* today blaming the media for stoking fears of a "second wave," which he says is "overblown." He congratulated President Trump on a job well done and attributed the rise in cases to increased testing, but there are ten states with their highest-ever positive rates, which means the virus is still out of control.

New cases in Oklahoma are also doubling, although they sit just above Oregon for number of infections. This is significant since the president still plans to hold a large indoor rally on Saturday despite everyone (except the Republican governor) trying everything possible to stop it.

A prominent opinion columnist in the NYT wondered aloud whether President Trump is trying to encourage a second wave since he is either oblivious to the virus or too inept to take any steps to protect the public. Supporters are already arriving in Tulsa to celebrate the reunion, waving flags and playing music. Maskless evangelicals will gather and stand shoulder-to-shoulder to hear the "the great White hope" insult everyone who does not bow to him.

JUNE 18, 2020

To give the future reader (my grands or great grands, hopefully) an understanding of the current state of our politics and how it intersects with the pandemic, a quick review of this presidency is in order.

Nearly everyone was convinced Hillary Clinton would win the presidency on November 6, 2016, since her opponent was a serial philanderer (seventeen women sued for sexual abuse), a failed businessman (five bankruptcies and dozens of lawsuits for breach of contract), with a history of White supremacy (starting with his father and their "White" apartment buildings) and a willingness to ridicule anyone with an opposing view. Trump's reckless speech and wild lies were continuous during the campaign; he appeared to be a pathological liar as well as a narcissist and a misogynist. He once boasted that he could shoot someone on Fifth Avenue and not lose any supporters. He could never win, we were sure.

But due to online foreign influence and an October surprise by James Comey, the Director of the FBI, Trump managed to narrowly win the electoral college even though he lost the popular vote by three million votes.

The three years and six months of his presidency have been even more disastrous than anyone imagined. America has lost its moral, ethical, and political standing in the world and now—due to federal incompetence—we are sick and dying as well.

The presidency is in crisis and so is the country. The pandemic is out of control, with twenty states now reporting rapidly increasing infection rates. The police brutality protests continue, and a second

Black man was killed by police without cause in less than a month. There are forty million unemployed workers and businesses are closing for a second time due to an increase in infection rates. Military and political leaders who have worked with President Trump are submitting articles and publishing books and declaring him "unfit for office." Hopefully, more Republican leaders will discover a spine and speak up for our struggling nation.

The Supreme Court just handed the administration a second defeat in a week, supporting protections for the LGBT workers and the DACA program for immigrants. Democrats are more than ten points ahead in the polls from the top to the bottom of the ticket with the 2020 presidential election just four months and three weeks away.

This president is feeling desperate which is why he plans to hold an indoor election rally in Tulsa despite an exploding pandemic. When asked about the risks, he told the press outside the White House that the pandemic is "dying out" and that wearing masks in public is a liberal political statement against him. And this is the man with the nuclear codes in his pocket.

Another 1.5 million workers filed new unemployment claims last week for a total of nearly 48 million people filing initial claims in the past thirteen weeks. More than half are still unemployed.

JUNE 19, 2020

There is a fundamental and dangerous problem with the way some Americans think. The independent spirit that led pilgrims across the Atlantic to escape the crown and sent settlers West across the prairie to claim a homestead has morphed into a demand for personal liberty that is devoid of a corresponding social responsibility.

A portion of our diverse population seems to feel threatened by "the good of the whole." They resent anyone telling them what to do and then demand the right to defend their opinions while armed.

They remind me of adolescents—filled with righteous indignation but devoid of common sense.

During the initial economic devastation of the nationwide shutdown, President Trump decided that stay-at-home orders were detrimental to his re-election chances and convinced his supporters that the danger had passed. He refused to wear a mask; didn't need a mask.

Now, not wearing a mask has become a political statement even though universal scientific studies show masks slow the spread…the only tool we have. The president's supporters refused—sometimes violently—and started a small but growing social media campaign that demonstrates how to burn your mask to "ignite freedom."

Dr. Fauci commented yesterday that the anti-science bias in the US is a disaster in the fight against the virus. The anti-vaccine movement is growing amid a pandemic that can only be stopped with an effective vaccine. Despite facts, those who support the president are against masks and social distancing and any sense that we are in this together. The virus, of course, is not political…and the virus is winning.

In honor of Father's Day, our adult children sent live lobsters from Maine, so we had a delightful and messy dinner with Hannah. We remembered another occasion nearly twenty years earlier when Michael was in D.C. for an internship and sent a similar feast home. Hannah was just eight years old and puzzled about why her brother sent live sea creatures across the country. "Are they pets?" she wondered. Now she sits with us at the same kitchen table and pores over her medical books.

JUNE 20, 2020

It looks like teenagers who are stuck at home—with school canceled, sports canceled, summer camps canceled—took the advice of a wise grandmother on social media and signed up for thousands of tickets to the Tulsa rally with no intention of going. The young people in this country are angry that the virus is destroying their plans. They face a year in limbo, with no jobs or school, and blame President Trump for messing up the virus response. They are a force to be reckoned with.

The campaign claimed that a million people signed up for tickets with 100,000 expected to show, so an overflow venue was erected at great expense. According to the Tulsa Fire Department, however, a final tally of 6,200 supporters lined up to hear a lackluster speech by a furious President Trump. A spectacular failure for him, but perhaps an indication that his supporters are more concerned about COVID than we know.

Or perhaps it was the six members of his Tulsa advance team who tested positive for the virus yesterday, or the frightening spikes in infection rates in a dozen states, or the fact that the CDC and every health expert in Oklahoma asked Trump to cancel the rally.

During his speech to six thousand people standing shoulder-to-shoulder indoors—a super-spreader event—he said, "Testing is a double-edged sword since you find more cases. I told my people to slow the testing down, please!" He accelerates the spread with an indoor rally and then wants to slow down testing to hide the results.

Everyone at the rally should isolate for fourteen days. Instead, they will return home and go to work and deny there was a risk. The current spike in cases has been traced to the Memorial Day weekend and the premature opening in the Southern states. The next spike will be in Tulsa and nearby towns—more hundreds sick and dying from Trump's self-serving cruelty.

JUNE 21, 2020

Cases are rising all over the country and elected leaders from every state are wrestling with economic health versus public health, with personal liberty versus social responsibility. So far, it seems that economics and personal liberty are winning. But it only seems that way since the virus is winning, and these twin pillars of American strength will bow once again to the reality of the pandemic.

Since there is no national strategy—besides denial—individual states are left to chart their own course, and since there is pressure to remain "open" it falls upon each individual to decide what risks to take.

There are one or two new cases a day in our isolated corner of rural Oregon. And there are license plates from two dozen states parked on main street in Joseph—from New York and Georgia and California along with all our neighboring states. Soon it will be four or five new cases a day and then ten or twelve.

We set up "Pandemic Beach" in the front yard with chairs and tables spaced six feet apart over a 30x30 gravel pad above the stream. There are tiki torches and a chimney fireplace, and a barrel filled with beer. We miss our friends and long for them to visit…safely.

It is hard to keep our distance from each other and I confess to hugging Hannah before she left. I also hugged my friend Marcy because she needed the physical touch of a friend. We were outside and turned our faces away and hopefully there was no harm done. Only amid a pandemic could we feel guilty for hugging the people we love.

But we are hungry for each other by design, so maybe when people demand we reopen the states, they care more about companionship after a long isolation and less about the economy. Unfortunately, some will pay the price with their lives.

JUNE 22, 2020

Despite missing loved ones during the pandemic, the country also seems perched on the edge of anarchy driven by selfishness. Public health officers are leaving jobs due to harassment and threats of violence against their families. But since President Trump doesn't wear a mask and has not canceled events and has told the country many times that the virus is going away, his supporters are increasingly angry because some businesses are still closed, and others require a mask. There are daily political attacks upon public health workers by a vocal—and sometimes violent—minority.

The European Union has seen its steep mountain-shape curve steadily fall and is preparing for the reopening of international travel on July 1. EU leaders are considering criteria for foreign entry from three countries where COVID is still out of control—specifically Brazil, Russia, and the United States—countries where the elected authoritarian leaders have downplayed the virus, and millions are sick and dying. For the first time in our nation's history, Americans are not welcome in Europe.

Nor are Swedes welcome in the neighboring countries of Norway and Finland due to their failed experiment to build herd immunity without a vaccine. They have 511 deaths per million which is even higher than the United States.

Unfortunately, our country has 5% of the global population and 25% of the global COVID cases—and the red wave has arrived. The flat plateau of cases we saw in April and May is now shooting higher with new cases in the thousands each day in some states. Our curve was never shaped like a mountain with a peak and a fall. When the blue wave subsided on the east coast the red wave continued to build steam. The disaster we anticipated in late March with tent hospitals in local parks may soon be visited upon the south and the west—a second wave.

JUNE 24, 2020

The Black Lives Matter protests are still going strong with an emphasis on bringing down the statues of rich slave owners and confederate leaders who were once glorified. Many of the tributes to confederate generals were placed throughout the south by the KKK during their resurgence in the roaring twenties—which was after the pandemic of 1918 and before the Depression of 1929.

Many states are passing legislation prohibiting excessive force and holding police accountable for the consequences of their actions. And it does seem that our country is more aware of how a racist history has integrated itself into our institutions and our laws and our minds. In this very bleak time, any change is heartening to see; we know society will never evolve as long as people judge each other from the outside in.

Social unrest has played right into the president's racist rhetoric as we witnessed during his Tulsa Rally and at the "Students for Trump" rally in Phoenix last night, where once again he referred to the "kung flu" and called the BLM protesters "thugs." Despite an explosion of infection in Arizona, Trump held an indoor rally at a megachurch where 3,000 young adults sat shoulder-to-shoulder without masks to hear him speak.

It is important to note that Tulsa was the only place in the country in the past three months where six thousand people have gathered indoors. And you could find no other place in the world this week where three thousand young people intentionally gathered indoors. Think about the visual: three thousand young adults sitting shoulder-to-shoulder for several hours without masks in a virus hotspot. It is difficult to imagine that any country will want any American to visit anytime soon. How great is that?

The hospital complex in Houston, Texas—the largest in the world—is near capacity at 97% full so they house new COVID patients in the children's hospital. In Arizona, cases reach new highs every day even though people are waiting thirteen hours in the hot sun for a test. Many people decide to just stay home and brave it out.

Hospitals will reach capacity in Utah within the month. In Florida, where thirty percent of the population is elderly, cases are rising rapidly with thousands more COVID infections every day. Although the governor blames increased testing and protests, the increase is from community contact.

Several studies show that protesters are not spreading infection since they gather outdoors and many wear masks. But the bars and restaurants, churches and manufacturing facilities are full, places where super-spreaders gather indoors. California, where so much of our food is grown, is seeing the number of infections in their agriculture community skyrocket by a thousand or more each day. Masks are now mandatory.

There were 36,000 new cases in the United States in the past twenty-four hours, the third day in a row for record high cases, a number worth keeping an eye on.

JUNE 25, 2020

Thirty days of protest for racial justice

The governor of Texas allowed the stay-at-home order to expire at the end of April and by Memorial Day cases began to rise and now the virus is out of control; the bars have been closed again and restaurants are back to fifty-percent occupancy. There were six thousand new cases in the last twenty-four hours and hospitalizations have set a record fourteen days in a row. One of the most alarming statistics is the positivity rate which is near twelve percent of all tests. The governor threatened to shut down again if the rate rose higher than ten percent.

In Arizona, the positive rate began to rise ten days after the state reopened on May 15. Again, when people heard "open" they thought "over," and behavior reverted to pre-pandemic norms. Even with recommendations to wear masks, few people did. One councilman held an anti-mask rally in Scottsdale and yelled "I can't breathe!" before ripping off his mask, mocking two public health challenges in one act. (There were anti-mask demonstrations during the 1918 pandemic as well…so much for progress)

The CDC is concerned that opening the bars and restaurants and beaches has caused a rise in young adult and middle-aged people becoming infected. Before Memorial Day, people under forty-five presented a minority of new cases; after Memorial Day, they made up the majority. Many are asymptomatic so there is concern that the infection rate is easily ten times what is reported through testing. If these assumptions are correct, the country will be overwhelmed by the end of summer; it is anticipated that another 50,000 Americans will be dead by October 1. There were 40,000 new infections reported in the past 24 hours.

There were another 1.5 million initial unemployment claims last week for a total of nearly fifty million claims in fourteen weeks; many millions are still unemployed. As the end of the second quarter nears, some speculate that the GDP will have dropped by forty percent April-June. Hopes for a quick recovery are waning which means the recession that started in February could evolve into a depression that lasts for years.

On another note, the plague of locust eating its way from the Arabian Peninsula west across Africa is leaving starvation in its wake. It is estimated that 300,000 people in northern Africa could die by the end of the year if there is no emergency plan to feed them.

JUNE 26, 2020

Over 47,000 new cases were reported in the US in the past 24 hours. Every day we break the national record, and yesterday there were new state records in Texas, Florida, Arizona, Georgia, South Carolina, Tennessee, Idaho and Utah. The pandemic is exploding in the US and the world watches in horror as the great American experiment in democracy fails the COVID test.

Nearly a dozen states have paused reopening plans, including Oregon and Idaho. In the metro areas the message to wear masks has finally been heard, but here in rural Oregon people crowd the boutique stores and specialty restaurants as if our little resort town is somehow immune. Rural communities are very conservative and refuse to believe the science.

President Trump no longer speaks of the virus, but the vice president did stand at the podium yesterday and offer a series of lies and misdirection. He answered a question about wearing masks by reminding us that the Constitution guarantees free speech. "Liberty!" The state tried to close testing sites in Texas, but local leaders refused. Trump is down fourteen points in the polls with the election just over four months away. Desperation fairly describes his behavior.

The economic situation is dire, with nearly thirty million still unemployed; an average of three million new weekly claims were filed for sixteen weeks in a row. Normal consumer spending is stalled which means people in the service industries are still not able to pay their bills. More economic pain is coming, and it will trickle—or maybe gush—from the bottom up.

The Denver Metro Emergency Network is holding on…but funding is harder to find. They have served 244,500 meals since March 18. There is no news on whether Michael's coffee shops will survive.

JUNE 27, 2020

Keith and I watched a well-produced fundraising appeal called *Global Unity: Unite for our Future*. Popular politicians from a dozen countries pledged millions of dollars for virus protection and vaccine research; a diverse group of star musicians highlighted the need for unity during this challenging time in the world.

There was an emphasis on access *for all people* to any viable vaccine produced anywhere in the world, with the story of Salk's vaccine for polio presented as a modern-day model. Salk tirelessly worked to develop a cure for that crippling disease, then gave it to the world freely, child by child, until everyone was inoculated against polio. He forfeited $7 billion by refusing to apply for a patent for the vaccine, believing the "people already own it." And it is true, millions of people contributed over a thirteen-year period, creating the March of Dimes Foundation to fund polio research.

We know there is a similar race underway to find a response to COVID, and we are reassured by the fact that every scientist with the skills to search for a vaccine is frantically doing so. If we have a vaccine this year, it will be the fastest scientific response to a global virus in the history of the world.

But once we have the vaccine, we need 70-80% of the population to take it before we can develop herd immunity and end the pandemic. In addition to reaching the remote places in the jungles and deserts of the world, we need to reach the remote thinkers—the skeptics, the anti-vaxxers, the religious fanatics, the conspiracy theorists—who are already ramping up tales of tracking chips administered via the vaccine.

Dr. Fauci has warned that even an effective vaccine can fail without enough people willing to take it. Thoughtless people can easily deny science when they do not live with the ravages of disease, a disease that might be cured if we do what health experts advise.

The battle against science has been a feature of progress throughout human history, but science usually prevails: Angry weather gods were replaced by those with studied predictions, mythical origin stories by celestial observations, flat earth fears by global exploration, bloodletting by germ theory and now, hopefully, a global virus will be defeated by precision vaccines.

In every case, science challenged long-held beliefs. Currently, we have a vocal minority afraid of vaccines; they believe the cure is worse than the disease. Of course, they have never had the disease—have never even been threatened by the ravages of polio or smallpox, thanks to vaccines.

Only a fool would refuse antibiotics to treat pneumonia. Hopefully, this irrational fear of vaccines will evolve and save us from the rampage of COVID…that is, if a viable vaccine is discovered in time.

JUNE 29, 2020

On Memorial Day—May 25—Americans in southern states remembered the dead by flocking to beaches and bars after nearly two months of isolation designed to stop the virus. Most moved freely without masks, crowding together without concern.

Now—one month later—the bars and beaches and hair salons and gyms and movie theaters are closing again in the South due to a wave of infections among those who gathered despite the warnings. In Houston, sixty percent of those now hospitalized are under the age of fifty; infection rates have doubled, and ICUs are overflowing with middle-aged Americans.

At a Senate hearing today, Dr. Fauci says that if our behavior does not change, infection rates will double again and there will be 100,000 new cases a day. It seems, however, that warnings from public health officials do not influence those for whom personal liberty is the highest goal. Every day we see videos of arguments because someone is standing too close or not wearing a mask or spitting or coughing at people in anger. Public health officials are still receiving death threats.

Europe has banned Americans from traveling to their shores, and no world leader would risk traveling to ours. New York—which has seen a dramatic fall in cases after aggressive action—now requires visitors from sixteen states to quarantine for fourteen days upon arrival. Thirty-seven states have rising COVID cases; seventeen of these states are posting new records.

Another holiday approaches: July 4, Independence Day. The president will attend a rally at Mt. Rushmore in South Dakota where thousands will gather to honor past presidents who are remembered for serving the public good. Organizers have already announced that no social distancing or masks will be required at this public event designed to honor President Trump.

Here in Wallowa County, the community Fourth of July event—which draws several thousand visitors each year—was cancelled due to the governor's criteria for opening: no gatherings over a hundred people in Oregon's Phase 2. However, the conservative county commissioners gave permission to a local bar owner to raise private funds and hold the event at the public park. How is this even possible? Personal liberty is becoming a public threat.

JUNE 30, 2020

	CASES	DEATHS	DEATHS/MILLION	DAILY NEW
WORLD:	10,577,756	513,186	66	174,264
US:	2,727,853	130,122	393	46,042

The new measure of American exceptionalism comes in the form of high infection rates leading to a new global record every single day during the past two weeks. Today it is 46,000 new cases; we hold the record on every measure related to COVID: total cases, total deaths, deaths per millions and daily new cases.

The surge in cases across the nation is now rising so fast, it is difficult to keep track. Fifteen states have record numbers with thirty-six states trending upward. In another twelve hours more states will be added with more record highs…just in time for the Fourth of July holiday.

In the two previous administrations—spanning sixteen years—pandemics were researched, and reports were reviewed regarding what to do when the inevitable happened. Plans for responding to pandemics included contact tracing, quarantines, testing, social distancing, and masks, plans that were summarily killed by the Trump administration.

In all fairness, the two previous administrations did not maintain an adequate stockpile of supplies recommended in their own reports. The failure of successive governments has led to a disaster and the CDC now says there is too much virus circulating in the US to manage without drastic measures.

And still President Trump told the nation the virus is under control and will just disappear. Again, he lies to the public and refuses to lead. As Keith said recently: "Nero fiddles while Rome burns."

JULY 2, 2020

Yesterday there were 51,000 new cases in 24 hours and today there are 57,000—with 10,000 positives in Florida alone. Like twenty-five other states, Oregon has also set a record for COVID infections the past three days.

Keith and I have agonized over a decision to attend the memorial service for our best friend, Marty Hamilton. The event was limited to family only due to the pandemic, and after thirty years of friendship we were included. But we knew his adult children were flying in from other states so we took food and wine to the family today but will not attend.

Marcy just called to report that her stepson from Phoenix woke up feeling poorly after an intimate dinner with family last night and went to the local hospital for a COVID test this afternoon. He was positive so the memorial is canceled, and eight members of Marcy's immediate family are quarantined.

The community spread in La Grande since the Lighthouse church outbreak has now reached dozens of businesses including restaurants, bars, and manufacturing plants. People are working sick, then going for tests and returning to work—still sick—while they wait for results. There are eleven new hospitalizations.

The United States is so far behind the progress of other nations fighting the virus, we are viewed with pity and have been humiliated in the world community.

Just to provide perspective, Florida recorded over 10,000 new cases of COVID among twenty-one million residents which is more daily cases than all the Asian and European countries combined—2.6 billion people had just 6,760 cases in the same 24-hour period.

The nations of the world are closing their borders to Americans as they look on in horror. We have led the world in science and technology for a hundred years, but we are failing public health.

JULY 3, 2020

For the third day in a row the US has over 50,000 new COVID cases—25% of the new cases in the world even though we are home to only 5% of the people. By the end of the 4th of July Independence Day celebration, we will have over three million Americans infected.

It would be glorious if we could celebrate independence from stupidity but that is currently impossible. So, we celebrate democracy—designed as majority rule—but since we are currently controlled by a minority without enough common sense to protect public health, majority rule is also a stretch. Minority rule feels as oppressive now as it surely did when the British monarchy ruled the colonies—senseless and self-serving.

In successful countries, strong national leaders immediately geared up testing and tracing, provided free access to health care, required social distancing and masks, and presented a unified message and example to their people—and they successfully managed the pandemic. Our nearest neighbor to the north, Canada, flattened the curve almost immediately and has less than two hundred new cases per day compared with our 55,000 cases and rising.

Our failure is not a surprise. Tonight, 7,500 supporters of President Trump will gather at Mt Rushmore to hear him speak about "liberal fascists"—his newest talking point for re-election. Those in attendance will not be social distancing or wearing masks according to the Republican governor of South Dakota. They will be exercising their "Constitutional liberty" to do what they want without regard for anyone else.

Michael launched the Lost City Market this week. The "Pay-How-You-Can" farmers market will be held each Wednesday evening on the coffee shop patio with vendors offering fresh fruits, vegetables, baked goods, and some prepared foods for sale or free depending on what neighbors can afford. Michael's new venture, in collaboration with Denver Metro Emergency Food Network, was featured on the front page of the *Denver Post* today.

JULY 4, 2020

It is fair to wonder why Americans decided to party instead of protecting the education of their children, why celebrating "freedom" was more important than reopening schools…from kindergarten to college. Again, it seems that personal liberty has a higher value than the public good.

We wonder how parents will return to work when their children are home from school; how we open the economy when so many are afraid to go out. Again and again in these pages, the lack of leadership during national celebrations precedes a predictable surge in sickness and death.

Too few have learned that for one person to be totally free another must suffer, that there is no personal liberty without equal responsibility for others.

July 6, 2020

There have been 262,858 new infections in the US during the first five days of July. Southern states are filling hospital beds so fast, there will be no capacity left in two weeks. Forty states have rising rates of infection and the supplies for testing are in such high demand that one official commented the competition among the fifty states is like the *Hunger Games*, a movie in which nine districts compete in an annual fight to the death.

The experiment in Sweden is not going well. In addition to having the highest infection rate among neighbors it turns out their population of ten million still has more infection per capita than we do—538 per 100k in Sweden versus 402 in the US. Their hope was that personal responsibility would be enough to protect their economy, but with the virus spreading so freely, people did not have the confidence to conduct business as usual. Their economy contracted by nearly five percent this year and their unemployment rate doubled.

For now, it seems, the virus always wins. The president of Brazil came to power with support from President Trump and has adopted the same irresponsible and ignorant attempt to wish away the virus—what he called "a little flu." Now this willfully ignorant president is sick with COVID and so is his country. Brazil has the highest rate of infection in the world—next to the United States—and they are catching up at a blazing pace.

Pandemic Beach was a hit last night. We fired up the tiki torches and the ceramic chimney and sat under the stars with mountain streams bubbling in the background. The tables and chairs are six feet apart with comfy cushions and individual tables for drinks. If our guests are retired and careful, it should be safe to entertain friends on the "beach" this summer.

JULY 8, 2020

Houston is a city in crisis, with zero hospital capacity remaining, and people waiting in cars overnight for a test. Hearing this, many people are just deciding to die at home, with no diagnosis, no healthcare, no medicine to ease their pain.

Mississippi state legislators gathered for a two-week, in-person session but did not follow public health guidelines, working indoors without masks or social distancing. So now there are twenty-six legislators infected with COVID and anyone who had contact with these Mississippi leaders must now be tested.

Arizona currently has more cases than New York at the surge. They do not have enough tests even though they have asked the federal government for more. Of the tests that have been administered, 26.83% are positive which is the highest positive rate in the nation… and perhaps the world.

Arizona reached their first 50,000 cases in 138 days—in a little over four months. Now they have a total of 100,000 cases just fifteen days later. Patients are being transferred out of state because all the ICU beds are full, which is not surprising since there are very few to start with: in one county, there are a total of eleven ICU beds for one million people.

The positive rate in Florida is 18.7% which means one in five people tested are positive for COVID. They have one in five hospital beds available as well, with a very large population of older Americans at risk of complications. The entire state may reach capacity in two weeks.

The same is true for the other Southern states that opened before controlling the virus: Louisiana, Alabama, North Carolina, South Carolina, Georgia, Tennessee, and Oklahoma all report thousands of new cases daily. Most of these states did not expand Medicaid under the ACA, so their rural hospitals closed, and few minimum-wage workers have health insurance.

In the past 24 hours there were more than 60,000 new cases in the US, but President Trump wants schools to open next month and is threatening to withhold federal funds for states that resist. Just like opening businesses too soon—a decision that created the current crisis—he wants schools to open before the election so he can claim victory over the virus. But he has sown the seeds of his own defeat... once again.

JULY 11, 2020

Nine of the ten largest outbreaks in the US since the beginning of the pandemic have occurred in correctional facilities where sick inmates occupy the same small cell with those who are not sick. In San Quentin Federal Prison—where they kept the virus at bay for three critical months—infections exploded after 121 inmates from another prison were transferred without any testing and the virus came with them. They now have 1,500 positive cases and are erecting tents in the exercise yard to house the sick.

New unemployment claims for last week were reported and 1.3 million people filed new claims last week, the seventeenth week with over a million new claims. There are still somewhere between twenty and thirty million Americans unemployed, depending on the database.

Michael laid off his entire Lost City staff with two weeks' pay. He realized there was no way to remain open without customers walking by, and most of the people in the neighborhood where his coffee shops are located either work remotely or are unemployed.

And there is no way to keep a food delivery service afloat when overhead outpaces donations, so next week Denver Metro Emergency Food Network will make their last deliveries. The Lost City Market will remain open through the summer since the "pay how you can" market is well received by those in need, and they have ample donations of fresh food.

All our children had to deal with loss this week. Rachel called her dad in tears to ask if Michael could "give her away" since she and Kevin decided to marry in an Aspen grove in Crested Butte—plan B—instead of rescheduling the plan A wedding they canceled in April. They hope to have a meal with friends from their "pandemic bubble" and reserved a restaurant's private tent; plan C is a picnic. Michael will be the only family from either side attending.

Hannah just found out that her first year of medical school will be held entirely online including the white coat ceremony and the welcome week activities. After dreaming and planning and studying for nearly ten years, she will now begin medical school alone in her bedroom with a computer screen for company…like a billion others in the world.

JULY 11, 2020

In San Antonio, young adults are having COVID parties to see if the virus is a hoax. When someone contracts the virus, they throw a party and hold a raffle to see who is the next lucky stiff to be infected. The first partygoer to test positive gets the prize money and a deadly disease. A thirty-year-old winner landed in the ICU, and just before he died he told his nurse, "I guess I made a mistake; I thought the virus was a hoax."

The cognitive dissonance between facts and beliefs—especially for those who support President Trump—is astounding but not surprising given how difficult it is for human beings to admit mistakes.

The pandemic hoax theory—that Democrats designed the pandemic to defeat Republicans—was circulated on Fox News in March and April and is still an excuse for millions of MAGA followers to ignore public health advice even after three million cases. With an exploding infection rate, public health experts say we should avoid socializing indoors this summer, masks or no masks which is difficult for people in the South because of the summer heat.

But even here in temperate Wallowa County people do not take the virus seriously. A local farmer entertained two friends from California at his home in early July. A few days later he became seriously ill with COVID, and all the friendly farmers they entertained had to quarantine for two weeks.

My sister in Arizona is furious with their governor who has taken very little action even though the hospitals are full, ventilators have been rationed, and refrigerator trucks are on loan to house the dead. Under the guise of "freedom," the rules for masking up are left to the mayors but all the bars are open for business.

My heart goes out to those in the southern states who are in crisis for the same reason: an active minority do not believe the virus is real and do not take precautions while retreating indoors to escape extreme heat, a perfect storm for spreading infection.

Here on the edge of the Oregon wilderness it is not as difficult to avoid COVID. We had a lovely dinner on Pandemic Beach last night with two couples from our bubble, retired friends who also stay close to home. As a party gift each guest was given a small glass bottle of hand sanitizer made from 89% alcohol and sweet orange oil. We sprayed our hands frequently and no one needed to venture indoors.

July 13, 2020

Imagine the bars, beaches, and restaurants across the nation being crowded with virus deniers while hospitals are overflowing with the sick and the dying and parents are agonizing over the danger of sending their children to school. What happens when young people party while their community burns?

Imagine President Trump constantly telling the nation that we are "doing very well, the best!" at controlling the virus when we have more than three million cases and 150,000 dead. What happens when campaign slogans are promoted as science?

Imagine what the world thinks when the most successful democracy fails to provide the most basic needs for its people: health, education, housing, food. What happens when the dark side of freedom—unbridled liberty—ascends?

How did this happen? How can we fall so far, this fast? I am having difficulty writing what I thought was a simple family journal documenting a new challenge when we are living in the middle of a dystopian reality, a surreal nightmare unfolding in real time.

The fruits of our experiment in democracy have been harvested and sold to the highest bidder, which caused decay, destruction, and disfunction on such a grand scale that self-righteous people now refuse to wear masks in the middle of a pandemic; they fight over a perceived threat to personal liberty while their friends and neighbors get sick and die. Who have we become?

The real danger of democracy has always been the "triumph of mediocracy"—the part dragging the whole down with fear, loathing, and conspiracy theories peddled by a few talented grifters. How far will we fall?

JULY 14, 2020

The Trump White House tried to discredit the most popular and experienced epidemiologist in the US, Dr. Fauci, because he has painted a very stark and frightening picture of the failure of our pandemic response—an accurate picture illustrated with the most recent facts and scientific projections.

It was a coordinated campaign: First, there were random rumblings about Dr. Fauci by WH aides; then they sent an unsigned opposition memo to the press citing his earliest statements that were eventually proven wrong as the scientific community expanded their understanding of the COVID virus; then a senior official published a scathing editorial in USA Today trying to discredit the nation's most trusted health advisor; then Trump retweeted a claim by a game show host that the alarm over the pandemic was an attempt by Democrats to make him look bad.

Dr. Fauci has not been asked to meet with the president or the Coronavirus task force in nearly two months; he has not been given permission to be interviewed on major news channels or attend White House or CDC public briefings. But Fauci has given interviews to major magazines and at public health conferences and medical school graduations that are covered extensively due to his credibility and popularity with the American people.

President Trump cannot stand being upstaged by a truth-speaking health official beloved by the public and trusted by six previous presidents, so he sends his sycophants to silence him. It has backfired, of course. In addition to unprecedented pushback by the media and the public and even Republican leaders, Dr. Fauci is finally speaking up for himself, wondering aloud why the administration would say such things since it only makes them look bad.

The administration also tried to kneecap the CDC, requiring that all hospital data related to COVID be sent to the Department of Health and Human Services (HHS) instead of the CDC. This obvious attempt to hide the facts was soon rescinded and the missing data reappeared on the CDC website within 24 hours.

History will study the rise and fall of this stunningly unfit president for generations, and the consequences of his presidency on the lives and livelihoods of the American people, not to mention our standing in the world.

JULY 15, 2020

	Cases	Deaths	Deaths/Million	Daily new
World:	13,684,075	586,210	75	234,681
US:	3,616,827	140,144	423	71,750

The population of Sweden is just ten million which puts their death rate of 553 per million ahead of every other nation besides three countries in Europe with high elderly populations and early community spread. (Belgium has a higher rate but they count all nursing home deaths.)

China would have recorded nearly a million deaths by now if their death from COVID was equal to Sweden's. China refuses to participate in the global public health community by collecting data and informing the world, so it is impossible to know the actual infection rate. China's COVID numbers are a fiction.

The US is the only developed country without a national health care system and the only country where health insurance is tied to employment. The lack of testing in the US—characterized by long lines and a long week to get results—means that the number of infections reported represents just a fraction of the actual spread in the US. Like China, our COVID numbers are a fiction.

JULY 16, 2020

The Coronavirus task force prepared a report on "hot" COVID infection states in the US and of the eighteen identified, seventeen are led by Republicans—mostly across the South where the president's support is strong—so the report was withheld from the public.

President Trump continues to bully Republican governors who take COVID seriously. One day after the president visited Georgia, the governor signed an order prohibiting local laws mandating masks and sued the mayor of Atlanta who issued a mandate anyway. It would be impossible to make this stuff up.

Despite the federal government insisting that states reopen schools, they have offered no plan and no financial assistance. Most red states announce schools will open next month…again with no plan. California has announced they will conduct online classes to protect the kids and the staff.

In one Florida county, 31% of children tested positive and still the governor demands they return to the classroom. The governor owes his election victory in 2018 to President Trump and seems to be paying the bill with the lives of his constituents. In Corpus Christi, Texas, eighty-five babies under the age of two have tested positive for COVID.

JULY 17, 2020

In just four months, over 140,000 families in the US have lost a loved one to COVID and in some families, two members have suddenly sickened and died leaving children without parents and parents without children. The magnitude of the loss is difficult to fathom and so is the lack of a national strategy to stop the illness and death.

Future generations will look back and ask why the American people put up with a government funded by tax dollars that did so little for taxpayers, and why Republican leaders accepted and mimicked a failed strategy from a failed president—the bigger question.

The testing capacity of the states is still stalled, but President Trump has said he will not sign a new relief bill that includes more funding for testing, tracing, supplies, or the CDC. One Republican who was finally compelled to push back has wondered aloud if there is any way to describe this action besides "attempted murder."

The first COVID death occurred in Wallowa County yesterday just half a block from my brother's new house. A sixty-year-old local man went to Portland for a medical procedure and returned home with the virus. He died at home, without treatment.

On a positive note, Marcy and her family are now over the quarantine and do not have any symptoms of the virus. She will join us tonight for dinner on Pandemic Beach.

Some take comfort in the low death rate as infections soar, but they forget that people can be sick for weeks and months before they succumb. With 70,000 new cases per day, the death rate will rise.

JULY 20, 2020

Here is an update on vaccine development:

Between 140-180 candidate vaccines are under development by scientists in every part of the world. With eighteen vaccines currently in human trials, there is hope that an effective COVID vaccine can be developed by the end of 2020 with distribution next year.

An Oxford team leads the pack with a vaccine that stimulated the necessary two-pronged immune response in Phase 1 & 2 trials: T-cells were activated in fourteen days and antibodies in twenty-eight days, with 100% effectiveness after two shots. The vaccine is currently in Phase 3 human trials with 30,000 participants.

BioNTech and Pfizer both have reported success in Phase 2 human trials of 1,000 people, and fifteen other candidates for a COVID vaccine are not far behind.

If all goes well, there may be an effective vaccine ready for production in six months and pharmaceutical companies are beginning to make plans. Questions about who gets the vaccine first and how much it will cost are being discussed by vaccine producers, non-profit organizations, and national politicians, but those interested in the world economy will hopefully put health first for a change.

According to the Gates Foundation newsletter, it usually takes five years to produce a workable vaccine but with so many scientists working on COVID, there is hope that one will be ready for production and distribution in 2021. Depending on the details—whether one dose or two is required, how much refrigeration is needed, how to reach eight billion people—we may see an effective global response in half the time usually required…which could be 2.5 years. There is no quick fix.

In the future, when we hear reports of a new virus spreading from human to human, the science being developed now can stop a potential pandemic before it races around the entire world, killing millions. Hopefully.

JULY 21, 2020

Today marks exactly six months since the first case of COVID was diagnosed in the United States on January 21. Today there are over four million cases and 145,000 deaths in the US, with 1,122 people dying in the past twenty-four hours from the virus.

And still there is no *national* plan to address the pandemic: no testing plan, no contact tracing plan, no supply chain plan, no continuing economic support plan (even though twenty million people are due to lose unemployment benefits and eviction protection at the end of the week), no school opening plan, no plan to bury the dead.

However, there is a White House plan to deal with racial justice protesters in Portland, Oregon: send in unmarked Federal troops in war fatigues and let them loose on peaceful protesters; film the violence that results and make campaign commercials. Then announce more troops preparing to deploy to other Democratic cities, incite more violence and make more television ads. Continue LAW AND ORDER tweets several times a day from President Trump's twitter account to his MAGA base.

Is the federal crack-down on peaceful protesters a campaign strategy? Are they fueling violence in the street to justify a possible suspension of our constitutional right to vote this November? The president is down fifteen points in the polls and becoming desperate. Is he unhinged enough to try and hold power by force?

The next six months will make or break America. The scenario unfolding before us has been used in other countries to replace a fragile democracy with an authoritarian regime. How fragile are we right now?

The most hopeful sign we have seen—besides the millions of Americans protesting police brutality over the past fifty days—are the mothers in yellow shirts with bicycle helmets and face masks, linking arms to create a line of defense between the federal troops and the protesters in Portland.

The "Wall of Moms," as they call themselves, held the line despite attacks by federal agents with tear gas and batons. Spontaneous chapters of this ad-hoc group—mothers who have pledged to protect the protesters—are forming in other cities as Trump finds more Democratic cities to target with federal troops; more ways to fuel his re-election campaign.

JULY 22, 2020

Keith and I have been married thirty-two years today. He braved the grocery store and brought home a dozen red roses and a loaf of French bread; I made him pear and pecan muffins. It is an amazing experience—to measure our marriage in decades—and we are both truly grateful.

Several months ago, a microbiologist named Dr. David Ho presented two charts with infection curves on a timeline and said that if we end the shutdown too soon, the curve will not flatten and will in fact rise again at an exponential rate. But, he explained, if we stay the course and remain at home, we can severely limit the spread of the virus and open the economy and the schools much sooner.

Alas, the cries to "open the states" began to drown out more rational voices and churches were packed on Easter. By May Day, a handful of southern states threw caution to the wind and rolled back all restrictions meant to slow the spread. By Memorial Day most states were open which caused infection rates to spike starting mid-June and by Independence Day, our fate was sealed.

Today, the White House task force coordinator, Dr. Birx, warned leaders in eleven cities to take aggressive action to stop the spread of the virus. Neither the press nor the public were privy to this warning although details of the call were released by those attending. Here are the cities Dr. Birx was trying to warn: Baltimore, Cleveland, Columbus, Indianapolis, Las Vegas, Miami, Minneapolis, Nashville, New Orleans, Pittsburgh and St. Louis.

Some say that if we shut everything down for thirty days, we could stop the spread and open the schools. Others say that with four million cases and less than half recovered, it is too little too late; only a vaccine can save us now.

JULY 23, 2020

Forty days of protest for racial justice

Two months ago, the CDC produced a set of guidelines for opening schools the White House refused to endorse. However, the guidelines were leaked, and it was clear that schools could not reopen without investing a significant amount of money and time.

Now the CDC has published a second set of guidelines that confirm what every parent knows: children need to be in school. They also advise schools not to open until their positive virus test rate is under five percent. In Florida the positive rate is twenty percent and averages nearly nine percent across the nation. Besides stating the obvious, the nation has no plan for re-opening schools. It turns out that White House aides with no medical background wrote the second set of CDC guidelines.

The White House still insists the schools are safe to open no matter how quickly the virus is spreading. Teachers are up in arms; they are filling out their wills…and designating various political leaders as their health care decision makers.

Last month President Trump moved the Republican National Convention to Florida from North Carolina because local leaders refused to allow a crowded celebration. And now the Trump campaign has realized they cannot hold a convention in Florida since the state currently leads the nation in COVID infections. The Republican National Convention will be closed to spectators.

The Wall of Moms in Portland was joined by "Dads with Leaf Blowers" to clear away tear gas. A new "Wall of Veterans" who reject the need for unmarked federal troops to control peaceful protesters also joined the front line. But the president's campaign strategy—called Operation Legacy—continues with additional troops sent to Chicago and Albuquerque; he also threatens Philadelphia, Detroit, Baltimore and Oakland, California, and other cities with Democratic mayors.

Texas had nearly two hundred deaths from COVID in the past twenty-four hours. Hospitals are overrun with twice the number of patients as beds in the ICU; people are dying in the hallways and parking lots, but the Trump administration offers no help…not even federal troops since they are busy elsewhere. The United States leads the world in infections and deaths—recording a million new cases in just two weeks—but the only response from the president is to use tear gas against protestors.

Major League Baseball started the season in empty stadiums, with cutouts of fans behind home plate. Eight teams took the field, first kneeling in support of Black Lives Matter and then speaking to the press about racial justice. Players warmed up in BLM t-shirts, wore BLM patches on their Jerseys, and the letters BLM were chalked on the pitcher's mounds. There were testimonials from coaches and players aired during commercial breaks and we felt an overwhelming sense that the nation might be paying attention this time.

Another 1.4 million Americans filed new claims for unemployment last week, the eighteenth week with over a million new claims and the first week since April with rates starting to climb. Eviction protection measures end tomorrow, and unemployment subsidies end next week but extension provisions were stalled in the Senate, and they recessed without reaching a resolution.

JULY 24, 2020

Hundreds of physicians and public health officers have signed the following letter asking political leaders to "Shut it down, start over, do it right." to save the country. I have included the letter in its entirety.

* * *

Dear decision makers,

Hit the reset button.

Of all the nations in the world, we've had the most deaths from COVID-19. At the same time, we're in the midst of "reopening our economy," exposing more and more people to coronavirus and watching numbers of cases—and deaths—skyrocket.

In March, people went home and stayed there for weeks, to keep themselves and their neighbors safe. You didn't use the time to set us up to defeat the virus. And then you started to reopen anyway, and too quickly.

Right now, we are on a path to lose more than 200,000 American lives by November 1st. Yet, in many states people can drink in bars, get a haircut, eat inside a restaurant, get a tattoo, get a massage, and do myriad other normal, pleasant, but non-essential activities.

Get our priorities straight.

More than 117,000 Americans had died of COVID-19 by mid-June. If our response had been as effective as Germany's, estimates show that we would have had only 36,000 COVID-19 deaths in that period in the United States. If our response had been as effective as South Korea, Australia, or Singapore's, fewer than 2,000 Americans would have died. We could have prevented 99% of those COVID-19 deaths. But we didn't.

The best thing for the nation is not to reopen as quickly as possible, it's to save as many lives as possible. And reopening before suppressing the virus isn't going to help the economy. Economists have gone on record saying that the only way to "restore the economy is to address the pandemic itself," pointing out that until we find a way to boost testing and develop and distribute a vaccine, open or not, people will not be in the mood to participate.

Listen to the experts.

Public health professionals have made clear that even after we've contained the virus by staying at home, in order to reopen American cities and towns safely, we will need:

Enough daily testing capacity to test everyone with flu-like symptoms plus anyone they have been in close contact with over the last 2 weeks (at least 10 additional tests per symptomatic person). We currently have only 35% of the testing capacity we need to meet that threshold. The more people get sick, the more testing is required.

A workforce of contact tracers large enough to trace all current cases. That's 210,000 more contact tracers than we had in April, but the number keeps going up as infections rise. Most states are far short of the number of contact tracers they need.

In addition, we need more personal protective equipment (PPE) to keep essential workers like health professionals, emergency responders, and grocery store clerks safe.

Shut it down now and start over.

Non-essential businesses should be closed. Restaurant service should be limited to take-out. People should stay home, going out only to get food and medicine or to exercise and get fresh air. Masks should be mandatory in all situations, indoors and outdoors, where we interact with others.

We need that protocol in place until case numbers recede to a level at which we have the capacity to effectively test and trace. Then, and only then, we can try a little more opening, one small step at a time.

You should bar non-essential interstate travel. When people travel freely between states, the good numbers in one state can go bad quickly.

If you don't take these actions, the consequences will be measured in widespread suffering and death.

We need you to lead.

Tell the American people the truth about the virus, even when it's hard. Take bold action to save lives—even when it means shutting down again.

Unleash the resources needed to contain the virus: massively ramping up testing, building the necessary infrastructure for effective contact tracing, and providing a safety net for those who need it.

Many of the actions of our government thus far have fallen short of what the moment demands. Mr. Trump, federal administration, honorable governors: we remind you that history has its eyes on you.

Sincerely,

Matthew Wellington

Public Health Campaigns Director, U.S. PIRG

Public Interest Research Groups

The growing list of additional signees can be found online.

* * *

Here is a letter published in *The Dallas Voice* by a man who thought the virus was a hoax, held a family gathering, and infected every one of the fourteen family members who attended. His partner's mother died.

* * *

I admit I voted for Donald Trump in 2016. I admit traveling deep into the conspiracy trap over COVID-19. All the defiant behavior of Trump's more radical and rowdy cult followers, I participated in it. I was a hard ass that stood up for my "God-given rights."

In great haste, I began prognosticating the alphabet soup about this "scamdemic." I believed the virus to be a hoax. I believed the mainstream media and the Democrats were using it to create panic, crash the economy and destroy Trump's chances at re-election.

And so, believing the pandemic to be a hoax, my partner and I hosted family members on Saturday, June 13. On Sunday, June 14, I woke up sick.

By Monday, June 15, my partner and my parents were all sick. That same Monday, my in-laws traveled to witness the birth of their first grandchild. They took with them my father-in-law's mother and one of my partner's sisters. That night my father-in-law became ill. Then my mother-in-law and their daughter began feeling sick. So, they cut their trip short.

Two days later, my father-in-law's mother got sick. The new mommy and daddy got sick, too. We all tested positive for COVID-19. Only the newborn was spared.

My father-in-law and I both went to the hospital on June 24. The virus had attacked my central nervous system, and the staff stopped me from having a stroke.

My father-in-law's mother was admitted a day later. On July 1, she died of COVID-19 pneumonia. The chaplain wanted the family to break the news to my father-in-law, and he learned how his mother lay on her deathbed and then drifted off without any family by her side, even though he was in the room next to hers.

On the day of her funeral, which was July 14, five more of our family members tested positive for the virus. That evening, my father-in-law was put on a ventilator.

You cannot imagine the guilt I feel, knowing that I hosted the gathering that led to so much suffering. You cannot imagine my guilt at having been a denier, carelessly shuffling through this pandemic, making fun of those wearing masks and social distancing. You cannot imagine my guilt at knowing that my actions convinced both our families it was safe when it wasn't.

For those who deny the virus exists or who downplay its severity, let me assure you: The coronavirus is very real and extremely contagious. Before you even know you have it, you've passed it along to your friends, family, coworkers and neighbors.

Tony Green, Dallas, Texas

JULY 28, 2020

More than 150,000 people have died from COVID in the past 150 days. And a recent study showed 78% of the COVID patients who later recovered had heart damage and lingering respiratory issues. Long Haulers who have been sick for months have a Facebook page where they trade COVID horror stories and offer each other support.

Infections are rising in twenty-eight states due to large gatherings and a refusal to wear masks. The "rugged American individualist" will be responsible for the death of hundreds of thousands of family members along with friends and neighbors.

President Trump continues to lie to the American people. He suggests masks should be optional, that testing is overrated, that hydroxychloroquine is a cure. A fringe group of medical professionals called "Frontline Doctors" say masks are no help and hydroxychloroquine is effective despite dozens of studies around the world showing the opposite. For some reason, this fringe group were granted a meeting with the vice president yesterday.

Today President Trump and his son retweeted a video from the group leader, Dr. Stella Immanuel, a physician in Houston who supports the use of hydroxychloroquine and says masks are unnecessary. She also supports conspiracy theories about alien DNA in drug treatments and the danger of sex with spirits via astral projection. When asked by reporters about her bizarre theories, the president doubled down: "I like what she says."

Obviously, we are on our own. Schools cannot figure out how to open safely although many will try. The economic devastation of thirty million unemployed low-wage workers who are behind on rent will soon become heartbreakingly clear, Homelessness will be the next epidemic.

COVID will kill a million or two before a vaccine is available and a quarter of the victims will be in the US. We are still exceptional with five percent of the global population and 25% of the infection and death.

JULY 30, 2020

	CASES	DEATHS	DEATHS/MILLION	DAILY NEW
WORLD:	17,463,497	675,963	86	287,343
US:	4,568,037	153,840	465	68,569

Unemployment figures for the past week have been released and for the second week in a row the number of new claims filed has risen higher, with 1.43 million American workers newly unemployed. For nineteen weeks there have been more than a million claims filed each week with tens of millions still unemployed.

In addition, Q2 gross domestic product (GDP) figures were released today, and the US suffered the largest quarter drop in productivity in history with an annualized drop of 32.9% between April and June. This was greater than the Great Recession of 2008; greater that the Great Depression of the 1930's.

There were 68,000 new cases in the past 24 hours and 1,400 new deaths—one death every minute—which adds to the concern that the pandemic is continuing to wreck lives and livelihoods. The stock market opened down five hundred points so far today.

Adding to the panic, this morning President Trump tweeted that due to the rise in COVID cases, the federal election scheduled for November 3 should be postponed. Although he has no authority to postpone a federal election, he stirs the fear (and for some the hope) that he will escape defeat in November if there is no vote. He is losing by double digits in almost every poll. The next one hundred days will be the most important in the history of the nation.

JULY 31, 2020

Hannah and her longtime friend and roommate Ruoxi are here for a long weekend before they go their separate ways after eight years living together. Hannah is moving to Lebanon OR to start medical school and Ruoxi is moving in with her boyfriend.

Having them here is not easy. What are the rules? Can we be in the kitchen? she asks. We need to work, so what rooms are available for zoom meetings? Can we use your hot spot? Am I allowed to open the fridge? Hannah lived in this house for eighteen years and six additional summers and too many holidays and vacations to count. The idea that she could not sleep in her room was too shocking, so I dropped the idea of using the trailer.

She wants a haircut before she starts school, so she scheduled an appointment even though Keith and I have decided not to risk seeing a hairdresser during the pandemic. "I'm sure it is safer here than in Portland," she says. For her, perhaps.

We try to explain that even our best friends do not come into our home now, but this is a foreign concept to these young women who live together and visit boyfriends every weekend. They are careful, with occasional masks and hand washing, but are their friends careful? Who does Hannah's hairdresser live with, socialize with? Do they keep their distance? Wear masks? Who was the client before Hannah? Am I becoming paranoid? A little.

Like most people, we would rather risk infection than deny the ones we love. We will do the best we can this weekend, go to the white coat ceremony in person next weekend, and breathe a huge sigh of relief after we finish isolation two weeks later.

This is the new reality, the consequence of our failure to be responsible for each other due to the corruption of the American Dream. You can still reach the pinnacle of success in America, but not if you concern yourself with those you leave behind.

Future generations—with the benefit of hindsight and considerable study—might figure out how we let this happen, how we allowed the destruction of everything we value, every ideal we cherished including our longevity, our innovation, our economic success, our model of democracy.

I would answer that we drank the tea of American exceptionalism after the Second World War and took freedom for granted because we "earned it." That we allowed unfettered technology to dull our brains and diminish critical thinking just when we needed it most. That we were intentionally divided along cultural and racial lines and pitted against each other by politicians and corporations who encouraged tribalism to divide and conquer...and collect more than their share of the profit.

Perhaps a pandemic is required for the ethics of greed to surface, for the morality of inequality to be questioned. Perhaps the pandemic has forced us to pay attention to the danger of reaping profit without requiring progress.

AUGUST 1, 2020

As cases soar—nearly half a million new cases in seven days—the pundits, health professionals and politicians have finally accepted that there will be no national response to the pandemic, and that states, cities, and counties must play "whack a mole" instead.

Cases are surging in the South, West, and Midwest due to a lack of response to public health advice. Here is the reality: shutdowns lower the curve; normal human behaviors raise the curve.

This reality is becoming clear around the world. After controlling the virus in early shutdowns, nations that lifted requirements are beginning to surge again, including Japan, Israel, Australia, and Spain, to name a few. Of course, no one comes close to the infection rate in the US—which is higher than Brazil and India combined—since we shut down later and opened earlier than everywhere else.

"Sources" disclosed that the White House had a detailed pandemic plan in early April but shelved it when it looked as if the damage was limited to Democratic states during the blue wave; implementing the plan would require tremendous effort and they believed the red states—their people—had been spared. Now the southern states have more infection than the original blue states because they have yet to abandon magical thinking and put on a mask.

We are not alone in our magical thinking. Today, 20,000 Germans protested masks and vaccines in what was called a Freedom Day march in Berlin. The "Don't tell me what to do!" chant sounded like the rebellion of adolescents and illustrates the next stage of development required before human beings acquire enough moral maturity to evolve as a species; enough self-discipline to survive.

AUGUST 2, 2020

President Trump continues to demand that all schools reopen this month or face federal funding cuts. The public health professionals on the task force, Dr. Fauci and Dr. Birx, have both said that schools should not reopen unless the positive test rate is below five percent.

Trump posts continuous tweets accusing these two lifelong public servants of betrayal, he recommends the use of failed therapies to cure COVID, and he insists that the US numbers are high because we do too much testing. He is losing his mind.

Meanwhile, a survey of the top 101 school districts in the US shows the following: sixty percent will have online instruction only this fall, seventeen percent will ask parents to decide between in-person or online instruction, twelve percent of school districts are offering some kind of hybrid option, six percent consider their plan a unique combination and six percent have no plan at all. There are no major school districts in the US willing to risk the health of staff or students to offer in-person school this fall. We missed our chance to put the children first this summer.

Some nations have been better prepared. The Saudi government developed a plan with a very strict protocol to allow the annual pilgrimage to Mecca—the Hajj—to be held this year. Instead of the millions who usually attend, they selected a thousand pilgrims between the age of twenty and fifty, required a two-week quarantine, tested them, trained them in social distancing, and monitored every step along the way. So far, there have been no infections.

In Europe, on the other hand, the young adults have become so frustrated with restrictions they spontaneously decided to throw caution to the wind and visit the beaches and bars. The leaders are urging restraint, but it seems the limits of isolation have been reached.

Perhaps physical restrictions are not as effective in battling an epidemic as the quality of information people receive. Studies of the 1918 pandemic show that seven percent of economic damage was caused by the shutdowns they implemented, and a whopping ninety-three percent of the economic decline was due to the lack of consumer confidence. A more recent study showed that people who primarily consume online news on Fox, Facebook and Twitter are more likely to consider the pandemic a hoax; those who watched regular news channels and read actual newspapers were not so influenced by conspiracy theories and misinformation.

August 4, 2020

It has been interesting and informative to read about the influenza pandemic of 1918, 102 years before the 2020 COVID pandemic. Then, as now, people rebelled against the mask requirements implemented to stop the spread of the virus. Then, as now, there was a continuous promotion of strange cures, including the recommendation that disinfectant be sprayed into the nose and mouth, that children take two daily teaspoons of baking soda, and the not-so-strange belief in shots of whisky that were only sold in drugstores due to the emerging prohibition mindset. There were no vaccines or antibiotics available in 1918.

Then, as now, the government closed bars, restaurants, barbershops, cigar stores and other gathering places such as churches and schools. During the "Spanish Flu" as it was called since Spain was the only country publishing information about the pandemic, the US experienced three waves over eighteen months, starting with a staggering four-month period from September to December 1918 when 300,000 people—whole families—died in their homes. There were never enough gravediggers to bury the bodies, and price gouging for caskets was common.

The government was ineffective and had no national strategy to address the pandemic because they were fully engaged in World War I. To raise support for the war effort, they limited information and facts related to the pandemic—selling bonds was more important than saving lives.

Due to the espionage and sedition acts in 1917 and 1918, the US press could not provide information that might harm the war effort, so people got sick and died of the virus before news of the threat reached them. Then, as now, there were not enough nurses or doctors to treat the sick and dying.

By the end of the 1918 pandemic, 675,000 Americans had died from the virus including whole families and entire towns. The total death toll from WWI was 50,000, less than a tenth of the causalities from the virus but unlike today, the war and the Spanish Flu primarily claimed the lives of young adults.

Then, as now, it does not matter whether political leaders are fighting a war or running a re-election campaign; people's lives are not as important as political ambitions.

AUGUST 6, 2020

There are more than a thousand deaths every day from the virus, and on some days the virus takes one American every minute. States in the South continue to see a surge in new cases and have reached 100% utilization of available ICU beds.

Schools in the South reopened on the first of August, and within a day (or two) they needed to isolate students or close again due to positive cases. Many large school districts have decided to offer online learning only, an unfolding of a knowing if you ask me.

Although President Trump has repeatedly said children are immune—or almost—people are beginning to realize the depth of his magical thinking. Twitter and Facebook have removed his tweets and posts due to his dangerous misinformation. Imagine, the president of the United State being censored on a social media platform for lying and putting lives at risk.

The motorcycle rally in Sturgis, South Dakota will be held as usual this weekend; there may be half a million motorcyclists descending on a town of 7,200 to gather in the restaurants and bars and gamble with their lives.

These rugged individualists ride noisy bikes down a parade route, some in costumes of black leather and fur, and helmets with horns. When interviewed, they recite familiar propaganda regarding personal liberty and freedom from the virus hoax and a laissez-faire attitude about fate, echoing Trump. "It is what it is," he said about the death rate in a recent interview.

New unemployment figures were released today showing 1.2 million new unemployment claims filed last week, the twentieth week with over a million new claims. The official US unemployment rate now stands at 10.2%.

August 8, 2020

Keith and I traveled eight hours to Lebanon, Oregon to attend a virtual white coat ceremony with Hannah for the medical class of 2024 at Western University. The eight-hour drive was pleasant until we reached the I-5 corridor south of Portland and sat in traffic for thirty minutes. Even amid a pandemic with tens of millions unemployed, and even after we detoured to back roads, we could not escape rush hour traffic.

We stayed at the Best Western just minutes from Hannah's medical school and were satisfied with the hotel's COVID precautions: Masks required on the premises, no daily maid service, and a "full breakfast" consisting of frozen sausage sandwiches to heat with a microwave in the room, various pastries wrapped in cellophane, small yogurts, and coffee pods. Everything was single serving size and distributed at the front desk. We stood on red shoe stickers placed every six feet throughout the lobby and waited for our turn to gather breakfast supplies.

Although the pace of life in the city seems mostly unchanged, there are a few signs that a pandemic is raging. Most people are wearing masks in stores, which makes commerce more anonymous and often less friendly. Some rebels still refuse masks even though it is clearly posted that masks are required. In Costco, one rebel was loud and angry and seemed to dare other people to challenge her. I assumed she was dropped on her head in infancy…and hurried past.

During the drive home we saw numerous public service announcements flashing on overhead freeway signs reminding drivers that COVID is still spreading, and they should wear masks and "give space." It was heartening to see that many of our fellow travelers had a mask dangling from the rear-view mirror.

AUGUST 9, 2020

We are home and have no intention of traveling again soon. Every step requires a decision: Where to eat that is safe, where to find a clean bathroom, what hotel is best, which friends to call for a visit… can we hug our daughter goodbye?

The US will continue to experience virus spikes until a vaccine is available. Even when presented with the stark choice between gathering in bars or opening schools—a metaphor for maturity—enough people choose the bar to make safe schools impossible. So now we do what we can to keep ourselves safe in a rural environment and we wait…for a vaccine or at least more common sense.

Part Two:
The Gathering Storm

August 11-November 13, 2020

August 11, 2020

Unfortunately, the United States has become the poster child for what not to do during a global pandemic. For example:

Do not depend on for-profit healthcare, or a system designed by different politicians in fifty different states with benefits tied to employment. The collateral damage of forty million unemployment claims in five months is that millions of people and their families are suddenly uninsured. Even when jobs were added back a million a month in June and July—hourly jobs in the service industry—most did not include health benefits. Families are being hit with hospital bills amounting to tens of thousands of dollars after a loved one dies.

Do not expect the beneficiaries of an economic system that falsely claims profit trickles down to share wealth with the millions of Americans at risk of starvation and homelessness. Billionaires do not exist because of their compassion; they exist because of the corruption of capitalism. Why is there no sick leave, no living wage, no daycare, no health care, no housing guarantee for the those who provide the labor for profit? The pandemic has laid bare the inequality and cruelty of unregulated capitalism and the stunning neglect of the American worker during the past fifty years—which left many without a safety net when they need it most.

Do not assume political leaders will respond for the good of the whole during a pandemic since many are only focused on holding power. Do not assume people will follow public health guidelines indefinitely, especially when the threat is microscopic and remaining safe feels like an attack upon personal freedom. Pandemic fatigue is real and creates the conditions for a second wave here and abroad.

But do hope for a successful global search for the solution, an innovation that allows us to do better next time. We learn best when we suffer most, acquire wisdom, and decide to change...and the entire world is suffering.

AUGUST 12, 2020

The November challenger for the presidency and his choice for a running mate, Former Vice President Joe Biden and Senator Kamala Harris, made their debut today and added hope—and a sense of humanity—to the election politics that have left the country sick and dying for the past five months.

They each spoke standing alone at the podium with no spectators or crowds after all precautions were taken in full view of the cameras. The podium was wiped down with disinfectant, the candidates entered wearing masks, took seats ten feet apart, and addressed the issues facing the nation in separate speeches. Afterward, they put their masks back on and stood together with their spouses to greet the nation as running mates for the 2020 presidential election.

It was historic because the candidate for Vice President of the United States is a woman of color with immigrant parents of Tamil Indian and Jamaican descent, the first Black American female candidate for high office in our history. And it was heartening to see these leaders act according to the public health directives we have all been asked to follow.

The current president has addressed the nation and the press from his private golf club the past three weekends, mingling with a crowd of his political donors—all without masks. He insists the virus is going away and all the children should be back in school.

AUGUST 13, 2020

There were 116,000 American casualties in the WWI, which lasted four years. In the past five months, we have lost 170,000 Americans to COVID. Only in retrospect will we understand the depth of the loss from the 2020 pandemic.

Here are the US war casualty numbers including average deaths per day:

Civil War: (1861–1865) 655,000—449 deaths per day over 4 years
WWI: (1917– 918) 116,516—200 deaths per day over 1 year
WWII: (1941–1945) 405,399—297 deaths per day over 4 years
Korean: (1950–1953) 36,574—30 deaths per day over 3 years
Vietnam: (1961–1975) 58,209—11 deaths per day over 14 years
Iraq War: (2003–2011) 4,497—2 deaths per day over 8 years
COVID: (2020-) 170,415—1,136 deaths per day over FIVE MONTHS

Imagine we were engaged in armed conflict anywhere in the world and losing 1,136 soldiers a day. Suppose we had been invaded by another country and they were killing 1,136 soldiers a day. Would we fight back? Would any American not do their part to stop the killing and defend the nation?

My friend wondered aloud why I spend so much time documenting this unmitigated disaster and I had a ready response: After seventy-five years of global leadership, this country has failed to provide any leadership at all during the greatest global threat since

WWII. I am documenting the failure in the hope that history will not repeat itself.

But it may be a decade before we recover our economic, political, and moral standing in the world. And really, all we had to do was wear a mask and stand a little further apart. How did such a simple sacrifice become too much to ask? How did we elect a president who refused to ask?

The 1.3 million American soldiers who suffered the ultimate sacrifice for this country might ask the same questions given the chance. I am writing for them…and for my children's children who will someday wonder how this pandemic brought the world to its knees.

AUGUST 14, 2020

Some wonder—only partly in jest—if a raging pandemic is part of President Trump's re-election strategy. Initially, he stated that the virus would go away in the spring and that drinking bleach might be beneficial. Instead of providing testing and protective gear for healthcare workers, he authorized the purchase of 30,000,000 doses of hydroxychloroquine even though health experts warned about serious side effects.

Then he complained that testing increases the numbers of cases, so we should not do so much testing. Sure enough, even the severely inadequate testing available has been slowed down significantly, with fewer tests and longer wait times for results which renders the tests worthless. With no testing, we are forced to stay home from work and school and church…and the voting booth?

At the same time, President Trump continues to make unsubstantiated claims that mail-in voting is a major source of election fraud even though there is no proof. Oregon residents have voted by mail for twenty-two years—the first of five states to conduct voting exclusively through the mail—and twenty-two other states have some form of absentee voting including the military which has used mail-in voting for eighty years.

This year almost every state is planning an expansion of absentee ballots due to the pandemic, which makes delivery of ballots and returned votes critical to the integrity of the election.

In June, President Trump replaced the postmaster general with a political donor who has no experience with the post office and serious financial conflicts of interest. Immediately, this political loyalist cut wages and overtime, fired twenty-three top executives, destroyed mail-sorting equipment and started removing public mailboxes from American streets. Every state recently received a letter warning that the USPS could no longer guarantee that ballots would arrive in time to be counted.

People on both sides of the aisle complained about the president's efforts to ignore the testing crisis while simultaneously destroying the post office. There are letters of protest, inspections, lawsuits, and a general uproar among those who are informed…and an army of activists working on all fronts to stop the president from sabotaging the election.

Will our republic survive this attempt to impose an authoritarian regime?

AUGUST 15, 2020

	Cases	Deaths	Deaths/Million	Daily new
World:	21,605,487	768,409	98	260,409
US:	5,529,789	172,606	521	53,523

Finally, some good news. Today, the FDA announced they will provide emergency permission for a rapid COVID test developed by Yale University to be quickly produced and widely distributed. Yale has made the technology "open source," meaning they released it without a patent. The saliva tests are highly sensitive, can provide results in three hours in batches of thirty-two samples at $10 per sample.

There is hope that this inexpensive rapid test will allow sporting events to resume, that it might also be available to the teachers who are returning to classrooms, to the bus drivers who are bringing students to school, and to the children themselves who would be spared an invasive nasal swab.

There is even hope that we could eventually use a paper strip to administer the saliva test, like a urine test for pregnancy. We need hundreds of millions of these tests per day. We need to test ourselves before we attend classes or go to work or enter a mall; we need a COVID test before we leave the house to visit a friend. We need an inexpensive test to use every few days until a vaccine can protect us.

If you are rich or well-connected you can already get a "rapid" test. There are private doctors with testing machines willing to set up a tent at the entrance of your event and screen guests for $500 each. There are tests for politicians and members of professional and college athletic teams; there are tests for movie stars and recording artists and for the incoming class at our military colleges.

But there are no rapid tests for the rest of us, not even if you are sick, exposed, or willing to wait at a free testing site for hours in the hot sun. And we still wait days or weeks for results, which renders the test useless.

We need to test everyone as often as possible as fast as we can. Only then will we control the virus, get back to work and save the economy; only then can we hug friends and visit family members without fear.

AUGUST 16, 2020

Stories from around the world provide insight into the patchwork of responses to the pandemic in various countries…and the deadly consequences.

Sweden—a country that did not lock down, did not mandate masks, and encouraged people to continue living as usual—has recorded a death rate in the first six months of 2020 higher than any recorded in the past 150 years. Their experiment in herd immunity did not save their economy but the restaurants and bars survived, and the children have been in school. It is also true that the elderly in Sweden paid the ultimate price.

Venezuela—a failing country—has no healthcare capacity, no medicine, and an already ruined economy that led to an exodus of job seekers. Because of the pandemic, 100,000 are now coming home but President Maduro has placed thousands in detention centers to shift blame from his comprehensive failure. Neighbors are encouraged to report neighbors who might be exposed or infected, neighbors who are then detained without care. Most people are afraid to seek help when they fall ill since having the virus in Venezuela is a crime. The reported death toll does not represent the true depth of their suffering.

In Brazil, the authoritarian leader who came to power with the support of President Trump, initially considered the pandemic a hoax and joined his supporters in large gatherings without a face mask during the first few months of the pandemic. After he and his wife contracted the disease, his message changed but it was too late for the people of Brazil. With 110,000 dead, they have the second highest death toll in the world and a raging infection rate, second only to the United States. They bury their dead in pine caskets in newly cleared fields on the edge of the city. A recent photo showing row upon row of rectangular plots has been seared into the global consciousness—an indelible image of the 2020 pandemic.

There are many Asian and South Pacific countries that have a good national healthcare system, and they knew to shut down early to control the virus. But the entire world has learned that once restrictions on business and schools are lifted—even partially—infection rates rise. Controlling the virus without a vaccine is a delicate and heart-wrenching dance…one step forward then one step back, and sometimes two.

The same is true in Europe, with infections rising in Italy, Spain, France and Germany. When the first wave struck, these countries immediately went into lockdown and emerged with a flattened curve. Now, with an attempted return to a somewhat normal level of activity, their cases are rising again.

Around the world, people in their twenties, thirties and forties refuse to limit behavior once restrictions are lifted. They are going to bars, holding weddings, and crowding beaches this summer in a risky attempt to ignore the virus and pretend things are "normal." Our lack of maturity as human beings seems to be trickling down. Soon, the youngest children will be ripping off masks and hugging their grandparents.

AUGUST 18, 2020

"Ring around the rosy, pocketful of posies,
Ashes, ashes, we all fall down."

According to historical sources, this European nursery rhyme—which I often recited as a child while holding hands in a circle with playmates—was written during the bubonic plague of the 14th century (1346-1351) and describes the ravages of the plague: the red and chapped mouth, herbs to cover the smell of infected lymph nodes called buboes, severe and frequent sneezing, and the high death toll (25-50 million) including half the European population.

This history comes to mind because the first case of bubonic plague in California since 2015 was reported yesterday. In the 21st century we know bubonic plague is a bacterial infection that can spread via fleas (originally called rat fleas) and is easily treated with modern medicine—antibiotics. But in the Middle Ages, the infection caused multiple festering buboes, high fever, black spots on the skin, and a fifty percent mortality rate.

The high death toll from the Black Plague, especially among the aristocracy, led to new ideas and eventually to the renaissance in Europe, the cultural "rebirth" of art and literature. There was economic progress as well. The competition to replace serfs led to wages and a better quality of life, a challenge to the old feudal system of indentured workers tied to the land. Initially, the aristocracy tried to resist this change but eventually there was revolution followed by two centuries of intellectual and cultural progress. Most people with free time seek intellectual growth.

It seems the feudal system has been resurrected during the last fifty years via vulture capitalism. For example, it was reported yesterday that 350 Chief Operating Officers—CEOs of major corporations—made an average of $21.3 million each last year, which is around $11,000 an hour by my calculations. By comparison, the average worker makes between $10-$15 an hour, a wage that makes it difficult to rent an apartment in any American city.

Here is one definition of the feudal system: *"Feudalism served its purpose by creating a system where the king would appoint lords that would appoint knights to appoint serfs that would be expected to work the land and fields in exchange for food, protection, and accommodations."*

After this pandemic, the current feudal system characterized by profound economic inequality will also be challenged when hungry people without homes or healthcare realize the "lords" who run the corporations and appoint the politicians are not providing "protection" from systematic poverty.

It is interesting to see how history repeats itself—in both politics and culture—following severe challenges. After the 1918 pandemic a new freedom movement arose known as the "flapper" era, described as "young women flapping their wings while learning to fly." This cultural shift was characterized by women with short hair and tight skirts who were ordained with feathers and chokers and felt free to dance in a "wild fashion."

In 1920 women also organized and marched for the right to vote, and exactly one century ago today the 19th Amendment to the Constitution was ratified, granting a woman's right to vote—another significant cultural change following a global pandemic that killed an estimated fifty million people.

This country will face daunting challenges during the next decade, challenges that require a cultural shift from the White male patriarchy embodied by our current president to a sincere and lasting embrace of diversity and economic fairness.

We need to invest profits in progress, to legislate with common sense, to restore respect and dignity in our relationships—a vision presented by an experienced presidential challenger and his female running mate during the Democratic convention this week. Hopefully, a post-pandemic cultural shift is in our future as well.

August 20, 2020

New unemployment claims climbed again last week with 1.1 million workers filing for benefits after just under a million the previous week. There is concern that these job losses are permanent, especially for those with less than a high school education, a quarter of whom have lost jobs for good. The economy has contracted by 10.6% in six months—the largest drop since the depression—and unemployment hovers at 14.7%.

In contrast, billionaires have doubled their money during the first six months of the pandemic due to very favorable tax laws enacted by President Trump in 2017—his first act as president. They also gained wealth from the first pandemic relief package called CARES that put an additional $3 trillion of taxpayer dollars into the economy to blunt the damage from the shutdown. And now—again—we see where most of it went.

The infection rates in Georgia are extremely high due to Governor Kemp's decision to open the state on April 29 with few restrictions. He is against mask mandates for political reasons and in favor of opening schools for political reasons...the same schools that were closed a second time two weeks later when infection spread through the crowded halls.

Georgia occupies the laissez-faire position on the public health spectrum with one of the highest infection rates and death rates in the nation. In two weeks, my niece will marry in Georgia and although they have greatly trimmed the guest list, they are still expecting a hundred people on September 19—hopefully, in masks.

In Colorado, Rachel still plans to elope on September 11. The bride and groom will hike a mountain trail in Crested Butte with a train of lace dragging behind and exchange vows in an Aspen grove. They have implemented plan C, which consists of a walk in the woods with friends who live nearby, including one who can officiate. A photographer-friend will document Rachel on the trail in her elegant white dress.

After a six-year courtship not even a lethal virus will stand in their way—or dampen the joy we feel for our daughter and her soon-to-be husband who has always been perfect for her. We look forward to the beautiful photographs and, hopefully, the first of many grandchildren…the ones for whom I write this journal.

AUGUST 23, 2020

A violent series of thunderstorms has sparked fires throughout the west. Rain and hail with a lightning flash every few seconds woke us during the night and caused a small fire in the forest nearby. The air has that distinct August haze we associate with wildfire smoke, so we started our emergency sprinklers and will run them every few days until it rains in the fall.

But this is nothing compared to what California is experiencing. The same storm system produced 12,000 lightning strikes in the same 72-hour period and started over 650 fires in dangerously dry conditions. Extreme heat advisories were issued for all of California a week ago Monday, with thunderstorms and dry lightning; a few rolling blackouts were needed to save the electric grid.

California is on fire. Fourteen thousand firefighters with 2,400 engines and ninety-five planes are fighting fires that have burned 1.2 million acres in CA so far. More than a quarter million people are under evacuation orders, but it is recommended they stay with friends and family instead of in public shelters where the virus can spread. There are three fires surrounding San Francisco to the north covering five hundred square miles and one has grown so big it is now the second largest fire in CA history.

More storms are expected this week. And then, on the other side of the nation, there are two hurricanes barreling towards Louisiana and Texas. Marco is expected to hit Louisiana with high winds on Monday and Laura will batter Texas with hurricane-strength winds on Wednesday. Evacuation orders have been issued with the same caveat regarding the shelters: Only head to a shelter if you have no other option.

On a side note—but a good example of indoor virus spread—a woman in South Korea visited a Starbucks for a coffee recently, but instead of taking her drink to go she removed her mask and enjoyed her beverage at a nearby table. Due to excellent testing and contact tracing, public health workers were able to determine that this woman exposed fifty-six other customers in the store that day, but all the employees tested negative because they wore face masks without complaint.

We are seriously far behind countries that have implemented a national testing and tracing strategy. South Korea has less than 20,000 cases with three hundred deaths at a rate of six deaths per million (compared to our 545.) The US is number one on the global list for total COVID infections and South Korea enters the register at number seventy-five...proving testing and tracing works.

AUGUST 25, 2020

The country is in the middle of school openings for fall term with either in-person, virtual, or hybrid instruction. The in-person option favored by working parents is subject to the same unfortunate truths that many have learned after bringing any group together indoors: The virus thrives when boisterous people gather under the same roof.

It does not matter if the victims are adults or children, are working or learning or playing, although the virus seems to favor play; it does not matter if they are attending a wedding or a funeral or a church: breathing the same air indoors is risky. In Florida, nine thousand children have tested positive for the virus in fifteen days.

There are dozens of stories about college students gathering in groups and breaking the rules as soon as they arrive on campus. In Alabama, 565 new cases of the virus were reported one week after students arrived. Colleges are shutting down, students are being expelled for attending parties, fraternities are closing...but the young people are still gathering since it appears they cannot help themselves.

As I reported recently, this is happening all over the world. The second wave in Europe is being advanced by the young adults who socialize in bars and restaurants, in dance halls, and on beaches. They are looking for mates, and mask rules or social-distancing recommendations cannot stop them from the biological imperative to partner-up.

The modus operandi for the unpartnered in the world is not "*live long and prosper*," as much as we admire Vulcan logic and maturity, but more like "*whatever will be, will be*" from the Dickens novel *Hard Times*, written in 1854. The modern expression is YOLO—you only live once. I was young and reckless once—hungry by design and seemingly invincible—and learned from experience that nature (almost) always wins.

AUGUST 26, 2020

While Dr, Fauci was in surgery for the removal of a polyp, the White House pressured the CDC to issue new guidelines for COVID testing which has left the public health community reeling.

Previously, testing was recommended "for all close contacts of persons with COVID," but while the nation's top expert was literally unconscious on the operating table, the guidelines were changed to imply that asymptomatic healthy people who are exposed to COVID do not need to be tested. This change caused alarm due to the high incidence of asymptomatic spread. If those exposed and/or infected do not know they are infected, they can become "super-spreaders" and the repercussions could be devastating.

This was another attempt by President Trump to repress the official count of COVID infections for political reasons. The pushback was immediate among health experts and the CDC director tried to clarify by repeating the lie that "anyone who needs a test can get a test."

The politicization of the pandemic has been thorough with claims that a vaccine will be available before election day, that the infection is going away, that it is safe to open the schools, that anything to the contrary is misinformation designed to make President Trump look bad.

Political leaders celebrated their success in speech after speech at the Republican National Convention this week pretending that 175,000 dead is good—better than two million—and ignored the fact that nearly six million have been infected and one thousand health-care workers have died providing care and several million will be COVID long haulers, people who take more than a year to heal. More than one supporter of the president has said with a laugh that the pandemic will be over on November 4—the day after the election.

AUGUST 27, 2020

Racial tension continues, with protests in some American cities being held continuously since late May, since the murder of George Floyd on May 25 for passing a counterfeit $20 bill. Some police officers seem to be escalating aggression against Black men and women...or perhaps we are finally paying attention.

Last week a Black man named Jacob Blake was shot seven times in the back at close range while trying to reach his children in the car. During the ensuing protests, armed supporters of the police and the president roamed the streets of Kenosha, Wisconsin. Conflict between armed vigilantes and those gathered to protest the shooting eventually led to the murder of two protesters by a seventeen-year-old White nationalist with a long gun and a perceived grievance. The shooter, Kyle Rittenhouse, has now become the poster boy for the far right.

Last night in Portland—after ninety nights of continuous protests against police brutality and racial injustice—a supporter of the president was killed. It happened after six hundred trucks with giant Trump 2020 banners drove into downtown Portland and shot protesters with paint balls and pepper spray. The shooter has not yet been identified but this escalation of conflict between Trump supporters and protesters for racial justice is a clear indication of the growing division in the nation and the high stakes in the upcoming election.

Last week there were over a million new claims for unemployment benefits, which has been the case every week but one since March. For perspective, before the pandemic the average number of new claims in a week was 200,000 nationwide. Currently, twenty-seven million workers are still receiving benefits and only 42% of the jobs lost due to the pandemic have been reclaimed. This is partly because 70% of the bars in Texas and 71% of the beauty salons in California are still closed. More layoffs and furloughs are looming in the airline industry this fall as well.

AUGUST 29, 2020

In Germany, tens of thousands of anti-pandemic protesters gathered at the Brandenburg Gate in Berlin to protest mandatory mask and social distancing requirements. Many were far-right protesters who are also anti-government, and some who claim to just want the "liberty" to gather without masks; they share a "resentful suspicion" of the government and the pandemic according to news reports. Eventually, some tried to storm the parliament building and three hundred were arrested. As in other European countries, cases are rising and governments have extended public health measures, facing backlash from pandemic-weary citizens.

In India, cases are also rising, and they have the distinction of reporting the highest single-day count of new cases in the world, topping the US record by several hundred. Initially, India controlled the surge with strict public health measures but like other countries, as soon as the new case rate went down, the country started to re-open for economic reasons; Indians thought "open" meant "over," a familiar story. People in India removed their masks, opened the markets, and crowded too closely together.

Brazil continues a slow and steady rise in infections and deaths due to a lack of leadership that resembles our own for obvious reasons. Bolsonaro—the "tropical Trump" as he is called—still retains the support of the poor who are receiving $111 a month to help weather the economic storm. The death rate is higher than the US by two points.

In Sweden, the experiment in herd immunity continues, with a flattened curve due to fewer infections and deaths. It is interesting to note they have a cultural practice of isolating the elderly in "care homes" and assumed this would protect them. But Sweden allowed people to visit until the end of March and this mistake is the reason their death rate is twelve points higher than the US.

I have reported before that this experiment in herd immunity came at the expense of their elders. But the experiment provides valuable information regarding percentages needed for herd immunity and how painful it would be to reach sixty percent. In six months with few restrictions, Sweden has only acquired a fifteen-percent positive rate in the population with over five thousand dead.

There is significant progress in the antigen tests that might allow at-home rapid testing. Four tests have been approved by the FDA and are now in mass production. The accuracy rate is less than hoped, but the ability to limit community spread should allow more people to work and socialize. The question in my mind is this: Will people quarantine after self-testing positive or will they ignore results and put others at risk due to a senseless personal freedom belief—self before others.

AUGUST 31, 2020

	CASES	DEATHS	DEATHS/MILLION	DAILY NEW
WORLD:	25,608,291	854,424	110	249,703
US:	6,211,796	187,736	567	38,560

To reach immunity, one must be willing to cut the sick and old from the herd. The animal kingdom does this without guilt, leaving the task to predators. But what of us—human beings who develop loving relationships that span generations? Are we willing to let a virus thin our herd to save commerce, to maintain public education, to allow people to gather and partner up? These are the questions the world is debating.

The director of the WHO says the herd immunity strategy—especially as it applies to the elderly—is "moral bankruptcy." And again, morality is a human construct that herd animals do not possess; they make no moral or ethical decisions when using instinct to survive. But in human society everyone counts: the life of each part contributes to the whole and the whole moves "we the people" forward.

Without a vaccine, at least two million of us must die to reach minimum herd immunity in a country of 328 million souls (a 65% infection rate with a one-percent death rate.) Since at least fifty percent of us have underlying conditions that provide fertile ground for virus infection, anyone with health issues would likely be culled from the herd.

Most health experts, including Dr. Fauci, have advised President Trump that the cost of herd immunity would be too high to bear, but his new advisor, Dr. Atlas, disagrees. He is a radiologist with no infectious disease experience who was asked to join the White House Coronavirus task force after bashing Dr. Fauci on Fox News. The president's new advisor believes that herd immunity is a reasonable goal, that masks may not be effective, that schools should all be open since children don't spread the virus, and that college sports should resume.

Dr. Atlas—referred to by some peers as the new misinformation vector—currently meets with the president daily and stands with him at press briefings. Dr. Fauci—the most respected infection specialist in the world who advised six presidents over thirty years—has not met with the president in months nor is he invited to press conferences. President Trump discounts Dr. Fauci's vast experience by stating, "I inherited him."

Many are hoping that Atlas is right. Iowa State College will allow 25,000 football fans to attend the season opener on September 12 in Ames Iowa, the city with the highest per capita infection rate in the nation at 8.3 per 1,000 people. The athletic director hopes that mandatory masks, socially distanced seating, and a ban on tailgating will keep fans safe...another experiment, but everything related to this pandemic is currently an experiment and in addition to science, we also rely on state-sponsored wishful thinking.

September 2, 2020

Both the CDC director and the FDA director have made recent statements that undermine the nation's confidence in the agencies that are charged with protecting public health. Unfortunately, any indication that federal agencies have been politicized can erode public trust during a pandemic. "What it looks like at this point is you have a White House altering public health advice to improve election chances to the detriment of American lives," said biologist Dr. Bergstrom.

First, the FDC made claims about the benefits of convalescent plasma that have not been proven. Next, the CDC changed guidelines for testing that seemed to support the herd immunity strategy favored by the president and his new advisor, Dr. Atlas.

Then, the director of the FDA, Dr. Hahn, suggested that a vaccine could be approved prior to completion of phase three trials by issuing an emergency use order. The medical community immediately responded that these statements risked fanning the flames of anti-vaccine sentiment just when trust in vaccines is vital to saving lives. The claim has been walked back by Dr. Hahn with an assurance that approval will not be politicized, and even Dr. Fauci confirmed that he still trusts the process. The major pharmaceutical companies pledge no politics and safe vaccines. We will see.

The CDC just sent a letter to states suggesting they be ready with a distribution plan for vaccines by November 1—just before the election. But when pressed, they admitted it was just a planning exercise "not" for political reasons. There are three vaccines starting Phase 3 trials in the US, but none have reached the optimal number of participants (30,000) or are near the point of recording results.

SEPTEMBER 4, 2020

It is two months before the election, and we are hurting in so many ways. The nation seems firmly divided between those who fear the pandemic and those who remain willfully ignorant; while some of us forgo weddings and funerals others gather in defiance of all data that indicates gatherings are dangerous. We are sorted into political camps according to views inherited by geography and genetics and whatever 24-hour cable news channel we generally watch.

People are already mailing ballots in North Carolina, and other states with early voting not far behind. An "October surprise" will have less impact this election season, since half the nation will vote by the end of this month.

This weekend is Labor Day, traditionally the final holiday before school starts, and already there are indications there will be large crowds at the beaches and lakeside towns, including ours. The US now averages 45,000 new infections and a thousand deaths per day and the prediction is that more than 400,000 Americans will be dead by January 1st if we continue along this path.

Infection rates are surging in a hundred counties that are home to colleges and universities. College football games will be played in empty stadiums—if they are played at all—due to the hundreds of COVID cases discovered in the first two weeks after students returned. Some are being sent home without refunds for gathering in unauthorized groups which seems harsh, but school administrators are frantic due to the toxic clash between public health and politics; school officials are unsure what to do.

President Trump's new Machiavellian medical advisor is advocating that schools open despite clear evidence that there will be an immediate surge in infections recorded a week or two later. There is no guidance, literally none, from the Secretary of Education in Washington, D.C.

One college spokesman called it "national chaos," and it really is heartbreaking to see so many young dreams dashed. After planning and paying, packing and unpacking, college freshmen are walking alone on campus, anonymous in masks, required to stay in their rooms, kicked out for gathering in groups…and then packing again after a positive COVID test and a tearful call home. Will they ever forgive us for this unmitigated disaster?

Our higher education system is not designed to keep students apart, to house and feed them one at a time for two weeks, to provide care for those who become ill. But if they don't send a sick student home, what can they do? And if they do send them home, a campus surge could become a super-spreader event, potentially infecting families across the nation.

We are in a "damned if we do and damned if we don't" educational crisis that might have been avoided with competent national leadership. Our students are paying the price, including Hannah who attends medical school alone in her room, with online lectures and difficult tests and mountains of information she needs to learn.

SEPTEMBER 8, 2020

The West is on fire. The air in three states is deep orange from smoke and the trees are frosted with ash. There are hundreds of fires from the Northern Cascades in Washington state through Oregon to the Southern California border; there are ninety-six large fires burning in 4.3 million acres, setting historic records. Most were caused by lightning strikes and driven by high winds over the past few days.

Smoke is choking communities west of the Cascades, causing health concerns and evacuation alerts. Two small southern Oregon towns—Talent and Phoenix—burned to the ground last night and Medford, a city of 86,000, has been evacuated. There are several fires near Lebanon, and Hannah has been told to prepare for evacuation if the fires move any closer.

In Colorado, the temperature dropped from 90 degrees on Monday to below freezing on Tuesday with snow in the mountains above Denver. Rachel and Kevin just barely made it to Crested Butte before the mountain pass closed. They canceled the pre-wedding fishing trip because it is 26 degrees and snowing on the lake.

The wedding may move indoors since the trails will be muddy and cold on Friday with a high of 49 degrees. Hiking to the Aspen grove with close friends was plan C and now Plan D is a balcony at the hotel, with space heaters and blankets and face masks for their four friends—the remains of a once robust wedding party—and Michael. Wedding plan #A was scrapped for financial reasons and plan #B by the pandemic and plan #C is a victim of climate change.... which is causing raging fires and freakish storms in the West and the South and the East this year.

On another unhappy note, there are hundreds of new viruses being uncovered by melting ice in the Arctic—unknown viruses that have been buried for 15,000 years and could possibly be lethal to humans. The dance between climate change and coronavirus will define the next stage of life on earth and so we ask ourselves: Will the 2020 pandemic prepare us to respond without hesitation when new viruses appear? Will the fires and hurricanes and freak storms in the next few years motivate us to finally tackle climate change? Is it too late?

SEPTEMBER 9, 2020

Several months ago, a Columbia University study showed what would have happened to COVID infection rates in the US if mitigation efforts had started one or two weeks prior to the mid-March shutdown.

Closing one week earlier would have saved 36,000 lives and closing two weeks earlier—March 1—would have prevented over 100,000 deaths in the US. This is due to the exponential spread of the virus, especially with super spreader events where one infected person without symptoms can infect dozens who gather under the same roof.

The Columbia study is being cited again due to the release of a new book by Bob Woodward, a renowned journalist who has written dozens of books about US presidents over the past fifty years starting with Nixon who resigned because of reporting by Woodward (along with Carl Bernstein) on the Watergate scandal. The Woodward books about living presidents have made him a legend in his own time.

His second book on President Trump was released today, titled *Rage* and is based on nineteen recorded interviews with the president over the past year. Several of these conversations were held in the Oval Office but many were the result of late-night calls made by President Trump from his residence to the journalist without staff present or even aware of the calls.

One taped interview released today is a bombshell admission from February 7 in which President Trump warns Woodward that the virus is five times more lethal than the worst flu. He says he is playing it down to avoid a panic. "I like to play it down," he brags, and the panic of which he speaks is likely a stock market crash. He talks about the virus being airborne and very dangerous.

President Trump held six more rallies after February 7 (before the shutdown), packed events in which he told his supporters the virus would be gone by April; he said the Democrats were using the virus against him and that wearing masks was a way to make him look bad.

And still, Trump holds political events against public health guidelines and tells those attending to take off their masks. One hundred ninety thousand Americans dead and he continues to lie…usually from a podium on the White House lawn.

SEPTEMBER 11, 2020

Almost a million acres are burning in Oregon, 40,000 people have been evacuated, and 500,000 more are threatened by fire and ready to flee; five entire towns have burned, and thousands of homes have been lost to the flames. There is no way to count the dead. This is another once-in-a-century event on top of the virus, a "mass fatality event," according to the governor, the worst fires in more than a hundred years.

Never in Oregon history have the flames risen so fast or traveled so far in just a few days. Climate scientists and advocates warned that this would happen and indeed, hot winds raced down dry canyons west of the Cascades spreading fire so suddenly, some did not escape. Eastern Oregon—the drier side of the state—is prone to drought and fire but so far, we have seen no flames and very little smoke.

Today is the 19th anniversary of the 9/11 terrorist attack in New York City that left the Twin Towers burning and nearly three thousand dead on September 11, 2001. There were solemn ceremonies in New York as the nation once again mourned lives that were lost while the world watched in real time on live TV.

Our daughter was married in Colorado today under relatively sunny skies. We had a fifteen-minute zoom call before they took a short hike up Crested Butte to exchange wedding vows. We cried and laughed and wished them well.

SEPTEMBER 12, 2020

What the pandemic started the wildfires have finished: we are confined to our homes since being outside is now off-limits no matter how much space we have or how many masks we wear. The air is nearly unbreathable, even in eastern Oregon, with a thick gray fog of smoke wafting between the trees and a forest-on-fire smell that always causes high anxiety during fire season—the price we pay for living in the woods. We run our nine emergency sprinklers daily, like sentries surrounding the house to keep evil at bay.

The west coast has the worst air quality in the world right now, literally. Half the state is at the highest level of concern—extremely unhealthy: stay indoors—and since the wind is shifting, smoke is blowing east across the state. We have hope in the weather forecast: clearing skies midweek and rain a few days later.

Over a million acres have burned in Oregon, with twelve confirmed dead so far and dozens missing. The stories of personal loss are heartbreaking and so are the pictures of burned homes, parks, lodges, cabins, and all the natural wonders in Oregon where we gather for recreation—rivers, waterfalls, mountains, farms, valleys—have burned beyond recognition along the western side of the Cascade Range.

Hannah's medical student housing complex is surrounded by fields, a buffer from fires burning just a few miles north and south of Lebanon. The air quality is so bad, she needs an inhaler to breath. "Like smoking eighteen cigarettes a day," she said although she never smoked. So many students are sick from the smoke or have lost family homes or have been evacuated while attending online lectures that the dean cancelled tomorrow's final and gave everyone a passing grade. Hannah is driving home tonight.

SEPTEMBER 13, 2020

Taiwan is a country of twenty-three million people, connected by technology and a strong public health system supported by a testing and tracing program that is unsurpassed in the world. They have recorded a total of 499 COVID cases and one death so far. Their former vice president is an epidemiologist, educated at Johns Hopkins Medical Center, and he took charge at the very beginning of the pandemic. Everyone is connected by phone with the health services, and anyone with contact to a virus-positive person is required to self-quarantine for fourteen days. The health service knows if you are not in compliance via your phone, another testing and tracing success story.

As you can see, the failure of the US is difficult to compare to Taiwan due to the nearly exponential difference in number of cases and deaths; Taiwan has succeeded by a factor of thousands.

They did not shut down businesses or schools, or restrict access to elders, and the economy is intact. They succeeded because 99.5% of those who encountered the virus and were required to quarantine did so—all 250,000 of them. There was no unchecked community spread.

In the US, some people throw punches when asked to wear a mask and super-spreader events occur routinely; college students who test positive throw wild parties, and President Trump crowds thousands of people indoors in defiance of public health. See the difference? Some call it negligent homicide.

We asked Hannah to get a rapid COVID test at the local clinic this morning so we could enjoy her company in peace. She is still sick from the smoke with virus-like symptoms, so the clinic was willing, but she tested negative, thank goodness. We are huddled together indoors and spontaneously hugging.

SEPTEMBER 14, 2020

	Cases	Deaths	Deaths/Million	Daily new
World:	29,436,547	932,446	119	242,721
US:	6,749,289	199,000	600	38,072

President Trump decided to tour the California wildfires. In response to an appeal for federal aid for climate change, he said, "It will start getting cooler, you just watch." When the official responded that he wished science agreed, the president denied climate change again, saying, "I don't think science knows, actually." And then he smirked. And the virus will be gone by April, right? Wink.

It is impossible to take this president seriously, a man who brags that he doesn't need to read anything because he "trusts his gut." He continues to put "foxes in the henhouse," creating chaos as a substitute for his lack of leadership. The poorly trained communications director at Health and Human Services (HHS) that the president recently installed is now tailoring virus information to fit Trump's escalating rhetoric. But after posting a delusional rant on Facebook accusing CDC scientists of sedition, this unvetted and untethered director was suddenly placed on medical leave. His assistant, a man with no credentials, left his job the same day after it was learned he demanded that CDC scientists run all briefing information through him for a political check.

Although these attempts to politicize the CDC diminish public trust, the scientific community still has faith in their career colleagues. All the CDC scientists and the CEOs of pharmaceutical companies have pledged more than once that no vaccines will be released unless, and until, they are proven safe. I believe them.

SEPTEMBER 16, 2020

Dr. Atlas—the Fox News pundit turned top presidential health advisor—is not just advocating a herd immunity strategy, he appears to be implementing it.

After Congress demanded to see what information the White House task force was sending to states, it was revealed that between August 15 and September 6 several states with Republican governors received new recommendations regarding statewide mask requirements. Initially it was suggested that all states implement a mandatory mask requirement when their rate of virus spread was at yellow alert. Then—a few weeks after cases exploded and the rate turned red—Republican governors were told to drop the mask requirement.

During a television interview this week, the president said the virus would go away without a vaccine when we reached "herd mentality"—meaning "immunity"—a Freudian slip?

The scientific community is pushing back on Dr. Atlas, saying a radiologist is not qualified to make recommendations regarding epidemiology nor is he following established scientific thinking on the subject. Just this week, seventy-eight of his colleagues at Stanford University published a letter warning that Dr. Atlas peddles "falsehoods and misrepresentations of science."

As stated before, to reach minimum herd immunity, at least 65% to 70% of the population would need to be infected with the virus and recover—215 million Americans. Since the current death rate from COVID has increased to three percent, this means we could expect six million deaths among the 215 million infected. The overly optimistic one percent death rate that suggested 2.1 million dead to reach herd immunity is now unrealistic.

Imagine a strategy for dealing with this pandemic in which two to six million American deaths is acceptable...even if herd immunity was possible. Health experts have said that it is "not yet known" if antibodies produced by the infection can prevent another infection. They have also said the virus mutates every two weeks, which negates the notion of herd immunity altogether.

The head of the CDC, Dr. Redfield, finally stiffened his backbone and spoke truthfully at a congressional hearing yesterday. He said we will need to continue mitigation efforts for another year because it will take a year before everyone has access to a vaccine. He said the best medicine for prevention is wearing a mask even with a vaccine because we know for sure a barrier works. His days as director of the CDC are probably numbered.

SEPTEMBER 17, 2020

So much is going on that I have missed reporting the unemployment figures that are posted each Thursday for the previous week. They have averaged less than a million in the past three weeks, but not by much. For the week ending 8/29 new claims reported were 884,000; for the week ending 9/5 there were 893,000 new claims; for the week ending 9/12 there were 860,000 new claims. Ongoing claims for regular state unemployment insurance and the federal pandemic assistance program combined are still around thirty million claims per week.

There is currently no additional financial support proposed by President Trump or approved by Congress. The supplemental insurance program and the stimulus payments have not been renewed but there is hope an agreement between the more generous Democratic plan and the less generous Republican plan will be reached soon… before the election. Foreclosures and evictions are on the rise as the unemployed are faced with an impossible decision to either pay for housing or protect their health.

SEPTEMBER 18, 2020

So far this year we have been through an impeachment of the president (December 2019), a seemingly unstoppable pandemic, wildfires, hurricanes, and a plague of locusts. We are engaged in the most divisive presidential election in history—a battle for democracy itself—with a steady drumbeat of accusations from the incumbent, Trump, that he can only lose if the election is rigged. Every agency of the government has been used to tip the scale in the president's favor and still he trails by nearly ten points.

Today, in the middle of the worst year ever, we lost Justice Ruth Bader Ginsburg to cancer—the beloved champion of women and equality who has been on the Supreme Court since 1993. Now, with only six weeks before the election, the president and the senate leader will fast track her replacement which is either a boon to conservatives or a threat to liberals depending on where you stand politically. The election has become even more divisive, which would have seemed impossible yesterday.

A friend who was feeling distressed about the election asked if I thought the results would be honored and we would have a peaceful transition of power—the hallmark of our democracy for 250 years.

"Trust the people." I said without thinking, "not the politicians." If we focus on the tricks and the lies and the corruption of power, we will see only misery. But our strength resides in the whole—in the people—and together we will move beyond the selfishness of our animal nature. Two steps forward and one step back is still progress... real human progress.

I will take my own advice and ignore the noise of the politicians who seek power for personal gain and remember that real power resides in the hearts and minds of the people.

SEPTEMBER 19, 2020

Today the head of Health and Human Services (HHS), Secretary Alex Azar, the umbrella over the CDC and FDA, announced that all rules regarding medicine, medical appliances, and vaccines must be signed by the Secretary of HHS. "Any prior delegation of rule-making authority, including the authority to sign or issue a rule or a proposed rule, is rescinded." The HHS oversees eleven divisions, including eight public health agencies and three human health agencies. The anti-science conservatives are celebrating.

This also means that the FDA is no longer responsible for signing off on the safety of a vaccine. This power—and many others—is now reserved for the president's political appointee and adds another major agency to the president's re-election arsenal. He now has control over the person who has control over releasing a COVID vaccine. Many have called this a "huge power grab" at a time when the country needs more trust in the FDA, not less.

SEPTEMBER 21, 2020

The end of the vacation season in Europe has brought fears of a second wave due to a high infection rate in countries that were hit hard in the first wave—France, Spain, Italy and the UK—countries that controlled the virus with lockdowns from March to June. There are protests in major cities against mitigation efforts amid fears that another lockdown will be necessary.

In Latin America, there have been more than 310,000 deaths, and the expectation is that these numbers will surge because people have resumed normal behavior despite warnings that doing so will cause more virus spread in populated cities.

People everywhere in the world are experiencing pandemic fatigue but without a vaccine the threat of infection will continue to grow. Public health officials are pleading for people to protect themselves, especially with cooler weather approaching in the northern hemisphere and indoor spread more likely. The pandemic is in full swing…and winter is coming.

SEPTEMBER 23, 2020

It is hard to imagine the extreme state of anxiety and panic that currently grips the US, but a review of today's events might help.

This morning the Senate Committee on Health held a hearing with the directors of NIAID (Dr. Fauci) and CDC (Dr. Redfield) and

FDA (Dr. Hahn) who were questioned on the timing and safety of vaccines, the political influence on COVID information, and the conflict of interest apparent in drug company execs leading vaccine development for the government.

Although the directors pledged science-based decision-making, there are too many examples of political interference at the CDC and FDA to believe what they say. There are now calls for Dr. Redfield to resign from the CDC because the premiere public health agency in the world is no longer trusted.

In addition, Dr. Birx, who heads the WH virus task force, is considering resigning due to the influence of Dr. Atlas, the herd-immunity enthusiast who whispers in President Trump's ear. All our health organizations are in chaos because the politicians and political appointees are peddling pseudo-science.

Dr. Fauci finally shot down the misinformation of Senator Rand Paul from Kentucky who questioned mitigation efforts and promotes herd immunity. "You are not listening," Dr. Fauci said, and then again provided facts regarding herd immunity and reminded Rand Paul that the infection rate in NYC, the city with the greatest number of infections and deaths, is only 22%. Herd immunity requires 60%-70%.

This afternoon the attorney general of Kentucky announced findings in the Brianna Taylor killing committed by police executing a "no-knock" warrant at the wrong home. The only indictment was for an officer who fired shots into the adjoining apartment, not for the wrongful death of Taylor.

Some have commented that shots fired at the White occupants next door were considered wrong, but the shots that killed the innocent Black woman in her bed were okay. Protesters in Louisville—who have been on the streets for 194 days seeking justice on her behalf—were angry and the police who feel vindicated seemed aggressive.

Unfortunately, two officers were shot and wounded that evening. Armed vigilantes roamed the streets to harass protestors who gathered in a dozen cities. Most of the protests were peaceful but once again tensions are high.

This evening, we watched in disbelief as President Trump answered a reporter's question regarding the peaceful transfer of power: "I've been complaining very strongly about the ballots and the ballots are a disaster. Get rid of the ballots and you'll have a very peaceful… there won't be a transfer, frankly, there'll be a continuation."

The implication of these remarks is that President Trump's campaign is planning to contest absentee ballots because an overwhelming number of people are choosing to vote by mail during the pandemic. These constant fraud accusations—repeated by the president, members of his administration, and online by Russian bots—are designed to delegitimize the election even if there is no evidence of fraud. President Trump knows that Democrats vote by mail twice as often as Republicans and he wants to void those ballots.

A supporting strategy currently in play is for Republican governors in swing states to void the electors due to "fraud" and select those more representative of "the voters," which means they can give the winning electors to the losing president. "The Supreme Court will decide, that's why I need the ninth justice to be seated now," President Trump explains, knowing there will be constitutional challenges.

It is not hyperbole to say that our democracy is at risk of being destroyed by a fascist authoritarian enabled by a minority party that has captured the Senate and the Supreme Court. The November 3rd election is not between Democrats and Republicans but between democracy and dictatorship. We need to panic.

SEPTEMBER 27, 2020

Forty states are recording an increase in new infections this week. Dr. Fauci warned us in August that if we did not get our infection rate under 10,000 a day before fall, we would be in serious trouble. The US currently averages 40,000 new infections a day…and rising.

The two top states are North Dakota and South Dakota where the positive rate is over 25% due to the Sturgis motorcycle rally held in August in South Dakota, the largest event since the pandemic hit the US. Four hundred and fifty thousand people descended on a town of 10,000 to socialize, parade their bikes, listen to music, and mingle shoulder to shoulder.

The state's Republican leaders did not impose any restrictions during the event, and there are no restrictions now. But researchers can trace the virus straight through the heartland of America via the phone data of those who attended the rally and rode with COVID back home.

In addition to the Sturgis spread, there are now thousands of infected college kids in North and South Dakota as reported in *The New York Times* (since the government is not keeping track of infected students of any age at any school). After contacting 1,300 colleges across the US, the *Times* identified 130,000 infected students in college towns since the beginning of the month. These unfortunate young adults have become the nation's foremost super-spreaders.

The public feud between the CDC and the White House is in full swing, with Dr. Redfield of the CDC accusing Dr. Atlas of the WH task force of filling Trump's head with misinformation about ineffective masks and the benefits of herd immunity. The president happily listens to Atlas, since he is holding re-election rallies all through the Midwest and the South where thousands crowd together indoors without masks despite local public health leaders pleading for them to stop.

The CDC is also politicized. Information on how the virus is aerosolized indoors was up on the CDC website for less than 48 hours before it was taken down without explanation. (Informed people might panic and avoid political rallies.)

But there is reason to panic about COVID. The infection is widespread in the US and Europe and Latin America, with thirty-three million infected worldwide. The global death toll is already over one million, with a million new infections reported every four days. The second wave is upon us.

Deniers say the virus will be gone November 4—the day after the election—and across the world, the weary gather to protest "the hoax." But in terms of death, even epic wars do not compare with the destruction of microscopic viruses traveling the world, killing thou sands at a time without making a sound. The virus is humanity's most lethal enemy and those who treat the sick and the dying—and dispose of the dead—plead with the public to believe it is real.

SEPTEMBER 28, 2020

New York City schools are opening for in-person instruction today with every student being tested upon entry. They are short-staffed due to the recent discovery of positive tests in 150 district schools but have instituted mitigation efforts they hope will limit the spread. Again, every decision feels like an experiment during a pandemic.

In Florida, despite over 700,000 positive cases and 14,000 deaths, the governor has opened all businesses including restaurants and bars at 100% capacity. It is surreal to see videos of packed bars and patrons with no masks, but Trump says we are "rounding the corner" on the pandemic and he has done a "phenomenal job" despite over 200,000 deaths in less than eight months. He gives himself an A+.

SEPTEMBER 30, 2020

	Cases	Deaths	Deaths/Million	Daily new
World:	34,150,561	1,018,211	130	316,134
US:	7,447,282	211,740	630	40,929

I could not sleep last night. I awoke at 3:30 with the name "Proud Boys" in my head. This organization is not a group of veterans or firefighters or civil servants who celebrate their service to the nation. No, the Proud Boys are a new and growing White nationalist military group that infiltrates peaceful demonstrations to build a profile as "patriots" and thereby gain followers; they are racists and fascist agitators who organize on social media; they are domestic terrorists pretending to be patriots; they are a male-only MAGA hate group.

I could not sleep because earlier in the evening during the first presidential debate, the moderator asked both candidates to denounce White supremacy directly, in real time, in front of the American people and President Trump could not. Instead, he suggested that the Proud Boys "Stand back and stand by." He was encouraging his own private militia (formed after his election in 2016) and indeed, the Proud Boys logo now carries those words—Stand back and Stand by—on an identifying patch and their ranks have swelled overnight.

I suspect this militia will be dispatched to serve as poll watchers on election day, a promise President Trump made to attack "widespread voter fraud" despite no evidence of fraud—not a shred of evidence—found by his own commission in 2017.

He is eight points behind in national polls and is implementing a scorched earth strategy to destroy election integrity and remain in the White House. The late liberal Justice Ginsberg was not even buried before he nominated an arch conservative to take her place on the Supreme Court; Senate Republicans hope to confirm this new justice in less than 30 days. The president has already said he will need Supreme Court votes in a contested election.

OCTOBER 1, 2020

The national response to the presidential debate was just as expected. Newspapers across the country panned Trump's performance, calling it appalling and unpresidential.

Republican states are surging with COVID. In Kentucky there were a thousand new cases per day on average this past week. In Idaho, virus cases doubled in four weeks and the hospitals in several areas are overwhelmed. In Wisconsin, there is a 22% positive virus rate, which tripled in three weeks, and waiting lists for hospital beds. Trump will hold two rallies in Wisconsin this weekend.

For the past two weeks the president's campaign events look like they were held pre-pandemic, with crowded venues and no masks. This week ninety-nine female Republican candidates for congress sat together shoulder to shoulder for a campaign photo…with no masks.

There were no masks at the White House press briefing, no masks at the rallies, no masks when they announced the nominee for the Supreme Court Justice seat, no masks worn by the president's family members at the debate. No masks. No masks. No masks.

It is not a surprise that Trump supporters do not wear masks. *The New York Times* recently cited a study by Cornell University that traced the spread of disinformation about the pandemic: Of the thirty-eight million articles they found that contained disinformation, 38% could be traced back to President Trump. He is the king of misinformation, the super-spreader in the White House.

OCTOBER 2, 2020

During the past week, Trump held rallies in Miami, Atlanta, Virginia, and Pennsylvania; he held a private fundraiser in Duluth and two more at his private golf courses in Potomac Falls, Virginia and Bedminister, New Jersey; he announced the nomination for SCOTUS on the White House Lawn with 200 guests, held a reception for Gold Star Families inside the White House; he prepped for and participated in a presidential debate.

On Wednesday we learned that the RNC chair who often travels with the president tested positive for COVID. On Thursday it was announced that Hope Hicks, his advisor and debate coach, also tested positive.

Also, on Thursday we learned that Senator Mike Lee from Utah was not feeling well but attended the Senate Judiciary Committee hearing to discuss the SCOTUS nomination and then tested positive for COVID. He did not wear a mask and spoke loudly for ten minutes to emphasis his support for the nomination. There were seventeen other senators present, most without masks.

We now know that a few days before the hearing Senator Lee attended the SCOTUS nomination ceremony without a mask and was shown hugging and kissing people. Sitting three seats away was the president of Norte Dame University who has also tested positive.

This morning the nation woke up to the news that both the president and the First Lady have tested positive for COVID and are quarantined in the White House with symptoms. Later in the afternoon, Trump was transported to Walter Reed hospital with moderate symptoms and rising concern.

After reviewing how many people with whom the president had contact this week, more positive cases among members of the Senate and the administration and the staff are expected. This is a worst-case scenario. We are thirty days from the election and two weeks from the hearing for the SCOTUS nominee, not to mention the national security issues we face if the US president becomes seriously ill.

OCTOBER 3, 2020

We find no satisfaction in the fact that President Trump was wrong about COVID and is suffering from the illness. He has been wrong for nine months—providing false assurances and misinformation—and many have suffered and died as a result, but there is only heartbreak for anyone who contracts this terrible virus.

The list is growing: In addition to the president, First Lady, president of Notre Dame, two senators and his advisor Hope Hicks, we now know there are others whose COVID tests are currently being confirmed including another Republican senator, and Kellyanne Conway, and ex-Governor Chris Christie who was also a debate coach. The SCOTUS nomination was a super spreader event, and the White House has become a hotspot for the virus.

We do not yet know if Trump's challenger, Joe Biden, was exposed during the debate since the timeline of the president's positive test is in dispute. He sent a tweet Friday morning that he tested positive, but his physician stated he was positive 36 hours before that; if so, he was positive Wednesday morning after the debate and before he attended another two full days of events. The most infectious time is the two days BEFORE symptoms emerge, so the safety of the debate is in question. Already, Cleveland has announced there are eleven positive cases related to debate prep.

At this point, the vice president, speaker of the house, chair of the senate judiciary committee, secretary of state and the secretary of the treasury should be in quarantine to guarantee a smooth continuation of the government. The attorney general has said he will not quarantine even though he was at the SCOTUS event on September 26. The vice president announced he will attend rallies in-person next week, but that could easily change.

President Trump was given an experimental therapy on Thursday morning under "compassionate use" authorization. The monoclonal antibody therapy is designed to stimulate an immune response to the virus. He will receive one dose each day for five days.

A WH spokesperson told reporters at the hospital that "the president is still not on a path to full recovery." The next 48 hours will "tell the tale."

OCTOBER 4, 2020

It appears the confusion over the timeline for the president's COVID infection is due to White House efforts to hide the fact that he attended a high-dollar fundraising event in New Jersey AFTER being exposed and/or testing positive and starting treatment. We do not know for sure when he first tested positive, but we do know he had two positive tests on Thursday. More than two hundred of the president's wealthiest supporters must now submit to testing and tracing.

We are still getting mixed messages about his current condition. At the daily briefing we were told that in addition to the Remdesivir and the experimental antibody cocktail, he is taking steroids to aid his breathing since he needed oxygen on two occasions Friday. His physician says he might be released from the hospital tomorrow. No one knows what to believe but according to various COVID experts, the days ahead are critical and Trump is not out of the woods by any measure.

There are now three Republican senators who have contracted the virus, and several others who are in quarantine due to exposure. The Senate majority leader has realized he cannot conduct any votes for the next two weeks—not on a stimulus package or for the Supreme Court nominee he is desperate to confirm. As it now stands the US Senate will have only fifteen days to confirm the arch conservative nominee, Amy Coney Barrett, before the November 3 presidential election, an election in which they may lose the Republican majority. The cost of recklessness regarding the pandemic is now coming due.

President Trump briefly left his sickbed this afternoon to drive by a few hundred of his supporters gathered outside Walter Reed Hospital. His motorcade made one circuit and returned to the hospital. The outrage has been immediate and widespread, captured by this comment from an attending physician at Walter Reed Hospital:

"Every single person in the vehicle during that completely unnecessary presidential 'drive-by' just now must quarantine for fourteen days. They might get sick. They may die. For political theater. Commanded by Trump to put their lives at risk for theater. This is insanity," Dr. James Phillips tweeted.

"That Presidential SUV is not only bulletproof, but hermetically sealed against chemical attack. The risk of COVID transmission inside is as high as it gets outside of medical procedures. The irresponsibility is astounding. My thoughts are with the Secret Service forced to play," Phillips added.

OCTOBER 5, 2020

The White House press secretary—who held press briefings Friday and Sunday without a mask—tested positive this morning along with two (now four) of her deputies and will quarantine for two weeks. So will the attorney general and other cabinet members and staff who have been in contact with the eleven infected members of the White House administration which now also includes the campaign director and the president's "body man." The president remains at Walter Reed Hospital.

Wildfires continue to grow in California, burning more than four million acres this season, double the highest loss ever recorded since 1933, the first year records were kept. This includes the August Complex fire which burned over one million acres in fifty days.

There have been a staggering 8,200 fires in California in the past three months, with 8,454 structures burned and thirty-one deaths. Seventeen wineries in Napa and Sonoma valley have been lost so far; the grape harvest was destroyed on the vine and wine cellars exploded in flames.

US stimulus spending ended October 1 and major layoffs have been announced, including tens of thousands of permanent layoffs in the airline, entertainment, and retail industries adding to the 4.5 million who have already lost their jobs. Five hundred movie theaters will close nationwide with a loss of 40,000 jobs. There are millions who cannot buy food, pay utilities or rent, and will receive no additional unemployment benefits.

In previous recessions, those in the top and bottom income brackets suffered a similar unemployment fate, but in this catastrophe the losses are almost entirely placed upon the shoulders of the lowest-wage earners—those in the service industry. Economists warn we are headed into the worst global economy since the Great Depression… but stock markets around the world are holding their own since the means of production are still intact.

The inequality surfaced by the pandemic inspired Pope Francis to comment on the failure of "market capitalism" and the need to provide an economy accessible by all. The title of his third encyclical—the most authoritative teaching from a Pope—is "Fratelli Tutti" which translates into "Brothers All," and includes both brothers and sisters according to a clarifying Vatican statement. Pope Francis also cautioned Catholics against becoming single issue voters. Interesting.

October 6, 2020

Over the weekend, thousands of gay couples posted photos of themselves in an affectionate moment—kissing—to the #Proudboys, successfully taking over the White supremacy hashtag with an object lesson in how to conduct peaceful protest—a stark contrast to the photos of flag-waving, gun-toting racists willing to bully their fellow citizens for sport.

Meanwhile, the Department of Homeland Security (DHS) just reported that White supremacists are "the most persistent and lethal threat within the homeland".

"I am particularly concerned about White supremacist violent extremists who have been exceptionally lethal in their abhorrent, targeted attacks in recent years," acting DHS secretary Chad Wolf wrote in a letter accompanying the report.

Last night President Trump was discharged from Walter Reed Hospital not because he was well, but because he insisted. "I feel better than I have in twenty years," he tweeted, and then gasped for breath as he entered the White House and removed his mask for a staged photo-op…twice. He still thinks he can beat the virus with bravado. Public health officials are aghast.

The medical community agrees that he likely has severe COVID pneumonia although the facts have been withheld from the public. The most dangerous time for this diagnosis is 7-10 days from first symptoms so he may be out of the woods in another five days. On the other hand, he may join the ranks of the hundreds of thousands of Americans who have been disabled by the disease or succumbed to it.

Today, the chairman and six members of the Joint Chiefs of Staff entered quarantine due to exposure from the vice commandant of the US Coast Guard who tested positive for COVID. In addition, the president's top advisor/ speech writer announced a positive test today and is in isolation at home. No one in the government has lost a job because of COVID.

The FDA submitted vaccine approval guidelines that require a two-month waiting period to monitor side effects before the vaccine becomes available to the public. The White House promptly blocked the guidelines since they did not meet the November 3 election timeline and then quickly reversed the block due to unfavorable optics.

President Trump abruptly ended ongoing negotiations for a second stimulus package with a tweet: "The negotiations are over." He said he will authorize a "big stimulus bill" after he wins the election.

His opponent is now polling between twelve and sixteen points ahead; it appears Trump's debate performance did not go over well with the American people. Seventy percent of Americans polled do not believe anything he says about the COVID virus. Twenty percent of Republican voters over the age of sixty-five have stated they no longer support the president. Four weeks to go.

OCTOBER 7, 2020

There is a question about whether Trump was positive for the virus during the first debate or during the SCOTUS Rose Garden event. The White House physician will not tell the American people when the president last tested negative for the virus; he refuses no matter how many reporters ask the question because the president does not want that detail discussed. "He was tested every day," his physician said to deflect the question.

Although President Trump and his senior advisors have always said he is tested daily, due to the spotlight on the White House outbreak, those same officials have finally admitted that he has not been tested every day. This may explain why the White House has refused the CDC offer of expert help with contract tracing. They would need to know the date of the president's last negative test to rule in or to rule out who needs to quarantine. The media calls President Trump's behavior "reckless."

But the damage has been done. Although the White House will not allow contract tracing, the news media has compiled information regarding how many people were in the path of the president and his advisors in the week before testing positive. It is estimated that six thousand people were put at risk of infection during the rallies, meetings, and events after the SCOTUS super-spreader event.

And if anyone needs more reason to avoid indoor spaces with those not in the immediate family, look no further than the president's debate prep team. As of today, six of eight close advisors who served in that capacity are currently sick with the virus. The White House has become a virus hot spot and a deadly ghost town, with most staffers working from home. So far, thirty members of the president's staff have been infected.

OCTOBER 8, 2020

Unemployment claims for the past week were reported with 840,000 filing new claims. The overall unemployment rate for September was 7.9%, which is double the rate in January before the pandemic; nearly thirteen million people are still out of work. Since more than half the jobs lost will not come back due to the impact of COVID on small business, travel, and entertainment, millions may be out of work indefinitely.

The economic fallout from prolonged unemployment continues. Many of the unemployed have lost their healthcare in the middle of a pandemic; many are responsible for large utility bills that were postponed but are now coming due. There are twenty-two million Americans with food insecurity, and nearly a third face eviction or foreclosure. According to economists, the damage from the unemployment crisis could be catastrophic for the American economy for years to come.

It does not look like there will be another stimulus bill before the election, and if the president loses, he is unlikely to sign a bill after.

OCTOBER 9, 2020

Oregon Governor Kate Brown (D) was recently under a recall threat for imposing COVID restrictions, but according to the data she is doing well controlling the virus. Oregon ranks 48th in deaths per million (138)—with Hawaii (115) and Alaska (81) at the number 49th and 50th positions nationwide. Here in Wallowa County, we have had thirty-six positive tests and one death, with no current hospitalizations or school infections.

Michigan Governor Gretchen Whitmer (D) also faced a recall threat due to COVID restrictions and then a state capitol invasion by armed militia and now a kidnapping threat. Thirteen militia members have been arrested for plotting to seize the governor and overthrow the government and are in jail on domestic terrorism charges. After the "LIBERATE Michigan" tweet from President Trump last April, we were warned that attacks by White male militias would be on the rise, especially against women with power.

Wisconsin Governor Tony Evers (D) implemented new restrictions last week to combat the worst surge in the nation, with an average of 3,000 new cases per day and a 20% positive testing rate. Hospitalizations tripled in a week, so they constructed a 530-bed field hospital at the state fairgrounds to handle the shortage.

Due to warfare between the Republican legislature and the Democratic governor, Wisconsin is known as the "individual liberty" state with every attempt to implement public health measures met with court challenges and public outcry even though the entire state is colored deep red on the virus map. Today, a Wisconsin judge ruled that the governor's mask mandate can stand, which ends a conservative challenge and restores common sense.

Really, the only argument to make regarding adults who refuse to follow public health guidelines is a "failure to mature." Some people are in a constant state of adolescent rebellion against authority and push back regardless of the cost.

OCTOBER 10, 2020

Hurricane Delta is the second devastating hurricane to directly hit Lake Charles, Louisiana this year and is now battering the area as a Category 2 storm. Hurricane Laura hit the same area six weeks ago with the most powerful storm in 160 years. The current storm is named with the Greek letter Delta because the English alphabet of hurricane names has already been exhausted this season.

Hurricane Delta has dropped more than a foot of rain and left thirty percent of the state without power. NOAA reports nearly $16 billion of destruction from hurricanes, storms, and fires already this year. Experts cite climate change for these increasingly destructive weather events. The people in Lake Charles have absolutely nothing left.

OCTOBER 11, 2020

A professor of public health at the University of Minnesota predicts that sometime this fall or winter the US will surpass 70,000 new virus cases per day and lose over 400,000 Americans by February 1, 2021. "America is on a collision course with destiny," he said.

Without a testing program, the entire nation remains unprotected from an exploding second wave. There is still no federal mitigation effort—no consistent messaging, no universal testing program, no required contact tracing—and the White House has become a hotspot for infection. We are at the mercy of the drug companies who are racing to develop and market an effective vaccine.

We go on with our lives, some refusing to take any risk, some taking too much, and the rest of us weighing whether we can have an outdoor lunch, or a hot sauna with one close friend, or a game of dominoes on the deck…or have adult children home for the holidays.

The New England Journal of Medicine, a two-hundred-year-old publication respected globally by those in the medical community, published its first ever political editorial signed by every one of its editors, titled, "Dying in a Leadership Vacuum."

Anyone else who recklessly squandered lives and money in this way would be suffering legal consequences. Our leaders have largely claimed immunity for their actions. But this election gives us the power to render judgment. Reasonable people will certainly disagree about the many political positions taken by candidates. But truth is neither liberal nor conservative. When it comes to the response to the largest public health crisis of our time, our current political leaders have demonstrated that they are dangerously incompetent. We should not abet them and enable the deaths of thousands more Americans by allowing them to keep their jobs.

OCTOBER 13, 2020

On Sunday afternoon a Christian musician from California advertised a concert on social media to be held in downtown Nashville. He called it a "protest" against masks and promised there would be no restrictions. He filed no permits of any kind and his gathering broke multiple laws. Nearly ten thousand people showed up, without masks, crowded together to hear songs of praise. Again, it is fair to wonder about people who demand personal liberty without accepting any personal responsibility.

The surge continues: There were no ICU beds available in Oklahoma City last night, or in six Mississippi hospitals, and there is one bed left in Bismarck, North Dakota. For the third day in a row there have been more than fifty thousand new infections recorded in the US. There are tens of thousands hospitalized nationwide and nearly a thousand deaths every day. Dr. Fauci recommends we "hunker down," which is what half of us are already doing.

President Trump touts his own COVID miracle cure at a cost of millions of taxpayer dollars and says there is nothing to fear from the virus. He is holding rallies among those who agree and falling further behind in the polls.

And on the heels of his very expensive "cure," the White House publicly adopted a strategy of herd immunity supported by Dr. Atlas and the Barrington Group, a fringe group of libertarians funded by the billionaire Charles Koch who declared that the world should just let the virus circulate.

There were universal protests from the public health community in the US and around the world including this statement from Director-General Tedros Adhanom Ghebreyesus, World Health Organization press brief, October 12, 2020:

Herd immunity is a concept used for vaccination, in which a population can be protected from a certain virus as a threshold of vaccination is reached. Herd immunity is achieved by protecting people from a virus, not by exposing them to it. Never in the history of public health has herd immunity been used as a strategy for responding to an outbreak, let alone a pandemic. Allowing a dangerous virus that we don't fully understand to run free is simply unethical. It's not an option.

First, we were told by President Trump that it was like a little flu and would go away; then that hydroxychloroquine was a cure; then that drinking bleach might help disinfect the insides. Now Trump says that we should all get the virus to achieve herd immunity and brags that "the virus is no big deal."

Only those who watch conservative media believe the virus is no big deal. Those who study the pandemic around the world can see that we have an EPIC failure in the United States due to our lack of leadership. In China, the leaders follow a rigorous testing and tracing program; in the US, our leaders pursue a herd immunity strategy. The infection and death numbers clearly indicate which strategy works. Without a federal testing program, we are trapped in our homes; without contact tracing, the virus cannot be stopped.

I believe the presidential election on November 3 will send an unmistakable message to our leaders. Voting has already started, and people are willing to wait for hours to make sure their vote is counted. The intimidation and voter suppression rhetoric from President Trump has encouraged people to vote as early as possible. Including the mail-in ballots, more than ten million people have already cast their vote for president this week compared to 1.5 million at the same time during the last election. We have twenty-one days remaining to vote.

OCTOBER 14, 2020

According to *The New York Times* vaccine report, clinical studies continue for vaccine candidates around the world. There are nearly a hundred in pre-clinical development using animals and forty-five in clinical trials with humans.

Thirty vaccines have moved to the phase 1 trial with a small number of people. If the vaccine successfully stimulates the immune system, it moves to Phase 2. There are currently fifteen vaccines in Phase 2 with several hundred people of all ages receiving the vaccine to see if age is a factor in safety and immune response.

The eleven vaccines currently in Phase 3 trial each require 30,000 people with half receiving a placebo. To be successful, at least fifty percent of those receiving the actual vaccine must be virus free after two months. This trial also screens for additional side effects.

There are six vaccines currently in the limited group, a category for the Chinese and Russian vaccines that have been approved without completing Phase 3 trials. These governments are taking a serious risk but do not face the same public pressure for safety that exists in the West.

For example, China is approving vaccines for use on an emergency basis including 100,000 Chinese students who will study abroad. Medical workers have been given the experimental vaccine along with hundreds of thousands of people in UAE, Morocco, Peru, Argentina, Brazil, Russia, and other countries where governments are willing to broadly test the vaccine before Phase 3 trials are complete.

There are no vaccines that have completed all three Phase trials and gained US approval. There are two vaccines in Phase 3 trials that have been temporarily halted due to unexplained illness in two test subjects, which is a normal development. The speed and global scope of this race to develop a COVID vaccine is unprecedented in human history—vaccine development is a process that usually takes years to complete, if ever. There is still no AIDS vaccine after nearly forty years, only a cocktail of anti-viral drugs.

Despite a strict adherence to vaccine development protocol in the US (and Europe) public confidence in their safety has dropped to less than 50% due to Trump's repeated promise of a vaccine before election day. CEOs and researchers have all pledged to put safety above politics and most people still trust the scientists; vaccine confidence rises considerably when accompanied by the blessing of the most trusted scientist in America—Dr. Fauci.

OCTOBER 15, 2020

	Cases	Deaths	Deaths/Million	Daily new
World:	38,153,843	1,102,433	141	399,585
US:	8,216,315	222,717	672	66,129

Europe is in trouble. There were 700,000 new cases of the virus in the past week, an increase of 34%. New mitigation efforts have been put in place in France and the UK to control the spread.

There is a curfew from 9 pm to 6 am in France, affecting twenty million people in Paris and other cities. Bars, gyms, and swimming pools have been closed and fines are being imposed. In the UK, people are not allowed to meet inside with people who are not part of their households, and outside gatherings are limited to six people.

In contrast, few restrictions are being enforced in the US. Rules on the size of gatherings and the mandatory use of masks are ignored by Trump and his supporters. He continues to hold super-spreader events—political rallies for thousands—where neither the Secret Service nor his supporters or staff or family members wear masks.

He continues to downplay the risks of COVID and belittles Dr. Fauci in his public remarks. During a recent town hall, he was reminded that wearing masks could prevent half of the deaths in the next few months and asked if he would tell his supporters to wear masks? Apparently not. "People with masks are catching COVID all the time," Trump says.

As a result, the US is also in trouble. Infection rates in the US have reached the highest level since the July peak, with seventeen states reporting weekly infections higher than any week during the entire pandemic. Many of these states are in the rural communities of the Midwest—including Montana, Wyoming, Idaho, and Colorado—where the virus has infected more people in the past week than in the first five months of the outbreak combined. Wyoming did not reach the first one thousand cases until July but had one thousand new cases last week.

Another 898,000 new claims for unemployment were filed last week.

OCTOBER 16, 2020

There were a record 400,000 new cases of COVID reported in the world over the past 24 hours, led by the US which reported rates just a few thousand shy of the highest here since the pandemic began—71,687.

We are told to "hunker down" for the winter, with infection barreling toward us like a freight train. There is too much momentum and not enough willpower to stop the train.

OCTOBER 17, 2020

On August 7—the first day of the Sturgis motorcycle rally in South Dakota that attracted nearly 500,000 people from all fifty states—both South Dakota and North Dakota were recording an average of one hundred new cases per day. Since the rally on August 16, cases per capita in those two states have seen the highest increase per day of any state, reaching 800 daily cases this week. And the same is true for neighboring states: Wyoming, Minnesota, Montana, Wisconsin, Nevada… all have recorded steady increases in the daily infection rates since late-August.

When you add the increase in cases due to the start of school and the flu season and the political rallies held by the president in those same Midwestern states, there is an endless opportunity for COVID to gain steam and plow into us this winter with overwhelming force.

President Trump held eight rallies this week, with thousands packed together and few wearing masks. Republicans seem to live in an alternate universe, showing loyalty to the president by denying the pandemic. Even here in Wallowa County his supporters predict the pandemic will be over on November 4, after the president wins the election.

His base is shrinking, however. Seniors and the educated White voters are jumping off the misinformation train and minority voters are heading to the polls in numbers never seen before. Tens of millions of Americans have already voted.

Unfortunately, even if he loses the election the damage has been done. The cost of this president's incompetence will create an economic downfall that is four times greater than the Great Recession of 2008, according to Lawrence Summers, a leading economist from

Harvard, a loss directly attributed to the failure of the federal pandemic response.

We do not have enough testing or PPE to open schools or businesses without spreading the virus; we cannot see our friends or family without serious health risks. We are held captive by incompetence and ignorance, and 400,000 Americans will die before the country is able to correct course.

OCTOBER 19, 2020

During a pause in new infections this summer, Sweden took a victory lap for its success in flattening the curve using very few mitigation efforts; the elderly took a hit, but the schools, bars, and restaurants remained open, and Swedes went about life in their normal way while the rest of the world was in lockdown. But now Sweden is seeing a dramatic upswing (173% this month) in new virus cases among the general population and is forced to place limited lockdowns in some cities for the first time.

These results are in stark contrast to Sweden's immediate neighbors—Denmark, Norway and Finland—countries where mitigation efforts prevented much of the suffering and death. Sweden is the only nation in the world with a herd immunity strategy, believing that letting the virus move through the population would save the economy and cause an acceptable level of collateral damage. During a drop in infection rates over the summer, health officials exported reports of their success to other counties—most notably the US—despite a high mortality rate.

And now the radiologist from the Hoover institute—Dr. Atlas—is heading up the White House Coronavirus Task Force and advocating the same failed and discredited strategy of herd immunity, a strategy that has never been tried without vaccines, a strategy met with outrage by every reputable epidemiologist in the world.

So, it's no surprise that our pandemic response continues to deteriorate despite the surge in more than twenty-five states. The vice president's task force is in disarray and President Trump only talks with Dr. Atlas, who confirms the president's misinformation bias. Trump discredits Dr. Fauci publicly by calling him an "idiot" and limits his press access despite a high demand for interviews.

In the height of absurdity, Trump also insults his election opponent by accusing him of listening to scientists. He increases his anti-science rhetoric as his poll numbers drop. Some of his anti-mask and anti-science tweets are censured on social media, but he continues to shout misinformation to his supporters at crowded rallies in the battleground states. Some continue to believe that the mask mandate is tyranny; some threaten violence.

Nearly thirty million Americans have voted already, an increase of nearly 400% over early voting in 2016, with two weeks to go.

OCTOBER 20, 2020

The House Subcommittee on the Coronavirus released memos from the president's task force that were circulated to governors in secret and warned that thirty-one states were currently in the red zone, which means they had more than one hundred new cases per 100,000 residents in the past 24 hours.

The White House knew about this surge but ignored the information and scheduled rallies in many of those states. Trump continues to talk down the pandemic and says "We are rounding the corner" while public health experts warn that we are a week away from a "rapid acceleration" in cases nationwide. It is likely we will exceed our highest daily rate of 78,000 new infections before the election on November 3.

Unfortunately, even as positive cases are rising, testing rates are falling so the surge may be happening at a faster rate than we know. In addition, the CDC just released figures that suggest there have been

300,000 more deaths this year than usual, so it is also possible that an additional 75,000 COVID fatalities have not been counted.

Some call this the third and worst wave which may be true, but the graph of daily infections in the US looks like a mountain range, with peaks that can be correlated to national events and mitigation efforts in between. This is not rocket-science.

OCTOBER 21, 2020

The FBI held a prime time press conference to let the American people know that Iran and Russia have voter information and are conducting threatening email campaigns in addition to other election interference we have yet to discover.

Armed supporters of the president are setting up camp at polling stations to intimidate voters. The Republican senate is pushing through the most conservative female justice in the history of the nation just twelve days before the election in a process so hurried and contrived that Democrats on the judicial committee refused to sit for the vote.

Infection rates climbed by 34% over the previous week in the US, with 1,225 beloved souls dead from the virus in the past 24 hours. It is no surprise that millions of Americans are having vivid pandemic dreams. Last night I dreamed of being lost in a mall, wandering around without a mask, watching virus floating in the air like a red mist. I often wake from very realistic dreams where I am sitting in a crowded restaurant shoulder to shoulder with strangers… all of us without masks.

The president's supporters would laugh at my fear and sometimes I envy their ignorance. But the virus is changing the world, moving in waves of sickness and death and poverty into every corner…and this malign force is far from finished. I hope fear protects me and my loved ones and everyone else who listens to experts. Right now, fear is our friend.

OCTOBER 22, 2020

There were more deaths yesterday in South Dakota and North Dakota than in New York State. With a positivity rate for new infections at 35% in South Dakota and few ICU beds remaining in North Dakota, these Midwest states are facing a terrifying winter. Still, there are no mask mandates or restrictions to control the spread.

There was a 40% rise in hospitalizations in the US this week. Some Idaho hospitals are at 99% capacity and the first patients were housed in the Wisconsin field hospital this week. Fourteen states had more hospitalizations in one day last week than during the entire pandemic so far. Ambulances are being turned away from hospitals that have reached capacity.

Boston public schools were shut down with a mere 24-hour notice. There have been nearly 200,000 infections on US college campuses this fall.

Courts continue to rule on anti-mitigation suits, with some allowing business as usual and others upholding mitigation efforts. Besides political affiliation, there is no rhyme or reason to the rulings, but the consequences of gathering indoors without masks are the same in every state regardless of the various interpretations of law.

Cries of "Liberty!" do not protect us from COVID, and Dr. Fauci again reminded the one million Americans who do not wear masks that doing so could save 100,000 lives…maybe their own.

New unemployment claims were down last week with 787,000 people applying for benefits.

OCTOBER 23, 2020

It was a record-breaking day for the nation with over 81,000 new cases. Fifteen states had the highest-ever number of new infections in the past seven days, with North Dakota still leading the states in the per capita infection race. Of the ten hardest hit counties in the US, seven are in Wisconsin where the state Supreme Court just struck down the governor's limit on indoor gatherings. Record highs for deaths were also reported in four states.

The most troubling statistic for people like us living in rural counties is that most of the increase in infection rates in the past seven days have been recorded in counties with less than 10,000 people, mostly in the West and Midwest. Friends in the medical profession warned us today that the actual infection rate in Wallowa County is not being reported in a timely fashion; the data is three weeks behind. In fact, I know of a handful of people sick with the virus who are not being tested and whose friends and family are not in quarantine.

On a positive note, the FDA approved the use of the anti-viral drug Remdesivir, which has helped reduce the death rate in severe COVID cases. The two vaccines that were paused due to unexplained illness in two test subjects have been restarted and the hope is that one or more can finish trials and get FDA approval by the end of the year.

OCTOBER 24, 2020

Five members of Vice President Pence's staff have tested positive for COVID, including his chief of staff, senior political advisor, his "body man," and two staffers. So far, he and his wife tested negative, but people are suspicious and wonder why he continues to hold political events with no social distancing or masks. He responds that he is an "essential worker" like a fireman or ambulance driver, or nurse and he is not subject to CDC guidelines; he will not quarantine.

President Trump is holding several rallies a day in the hardest hit states with no masks or social distancing in the airport hangers where they are held. Some call these events "Death Cult Rallies" and there is great concern that these events are responsible for the surge in Midwestern states.

The Senate will hold a confirmation hearing for the new Supreme Court justice today without any further discussion or debate. This arch conservative woman brings the right-wing majority to six of nine justices. Concern for reproductive rights and healthcare is heightened; one case before the court could strike down the Affordable Care Act (ACA) which has provided thirty million Americans with health insurance for the past eight years.

The ten Republican states that did not adopt the ACA or expand Medicaid for low-income citizens are now facing a critical shortage of hospital beds since dozens of rural hospitals had to close without this critical federal funding. If the new justice joins with other conservatives to vote the law unconstitutional as the current administrations wants, young adults and those with pre-existing conditions—like COVID long-haulers—will suddenly have no health insurance and there is no replacement plan in the works. Many of the president's supporters live in those same red states, so it is a mystery why they favor his re-election, why they vote against their own interests.

Sixty million voters have already cast ballots with nine days left before the election, another record-breaking statistic.

OCTOBER 26, 2020

Brazil and the US have a lot in common lately, including twin leaders who have downplayed the virus and played up miracle cures that do more harm than good. However, their collaboration to diminish healthcare in South America has gone far beyond denying the virus and promoting hydroxychloroquine. According to *The New York Times* (October 2020) these two authoritarian leaders ended funding for 10,000 Cuban doctors and nurses who serve the poor in South American nations.

And now, five of the top fifteen nations for COVID infections are in South America—Brazil, Argentina, Peru, Columbia, and Chile—and account for nine million cases combined. Between North America, Central America and South America there are currently twenty million COVID infections, almost half the total in the entire world. Something is amiss in the Americas.

In other global news: Ireland has shut down the country for six weeks, Russia has imposed a nationwide mask mandate, and protesters in Italy and Spain demand freedom from new mitigation efforts and clash with police. France reported a quarter million new cases in the past week; the US reported half a million. All the lines on the tracking graphs for Europe and the Americas are heading up at 90 degrees. The virus is out of control in more than half the world.

OCTOBER 27, 2020

New cases in France, Italy, UK, Spain, Germany last 24 hours: 109,871

As the number of Covid cases in Europe and the US rise, stock markets are falling in Europe, Asia and the US. With no new stimulus measures in the works and hospitals at capacity, US investors are showing their concern for the long-term health of the American economy. Although not as dramatic as the March fall, the Dow is down 1,500 points in three days of trading this week—six days before the election—canceling all gains for the month.

There are still twelve million workers unemployed, eight million new Americans who have recently fallen into poverty, 100,000 businesses permanently closed, and 865,000 women pushed out of the workforce (compared to 216,000 men) due to the challenge of closed schools, the end of flexible service jobs, and a lack of childcare—family supports that were vital for working mothers in recent years.

On Friday, the third-quarter financial data will show a historic rise in GDP, but it will not make up for the historic losses the economy suffered in the first quarter of the year. And the gains do not reflect the winners and losers in the current economy—those who can work from home are doing well, those who cannot risk either sickness or bankruptcy…or both.

OCTOBER 29, 2020

According to President Trump's son-in-law, who has been his closest advisor, a new COVID strategy was rolled out in mid-April as part of a re-election strategy. And in taped interviews with Bob Woodward, May 2020, Trump told him there were three phases of the pandemic: the panic phase, the pain phase, and the comeback phase.

In the interview, Trump explains that he decided it was time for the comeback phase in mid-April and took "control" of the pandemic from the doctors and the scientists in a "negotiated surrender." This does coincide with press briefings and a daily barrage of tweets about LIBERATING the blue states. Armed militia took up the call and paraded around with semi-automatic weapons to reinforce the strategy.

These masterminds reasoned that if the governors were responsible for PPE and testing and tracing, the failure to control the virus would be on their heads. If the come-back succeeded and the economy recovered, they would win re-election. Against the advice of the CDC, they issued "Opening Up America" guidelines on April 17 and the pandemic became a partisan issue.

The infection rates are now off the charts. The president has held dozens of rallies since his own "COVID Cure," asking thousands of supporters to show their loyalty by crowding together and refusing masks. "Take em off! Take the masks off!" he yells to the crowds.

The red governors welcome him, and the blue governors seem powerless to enforce the mitigation protocols they have in place. But the results are clear: There is an 82% rise in infection rates in the counties where rallies were held, and a recent Stanford study tracked 30,000 new cases to eighteen Republican rallies. Former Vice President Biden, his opponent, does not hold unmasked events.

Of the nineteen states that do not mandate masks, all have experienced a rise in infections including these states with historic positive test results: South Dakota at 46.23%, Idaho at 35.63%, Iowa at 38.72%, Alabama at 28.17%, and Wisconsin at 27.17%. Overall, the US has recorded record-high infection rates during four of the past five days.

The only physician now currently advising the president is Dr. Atlas; the epidemiology experts have been sidelined. There are no Task Force briefings and no federal pandemic mitigation plans, and testing has been curtailed in several states, including Florida where some counties have only one site reserved for those with symptoms. The herd immunity strategy implemented by Dr. Atlas is the perfect rationale for doing nothing.

Most Americans are appalled, and it appears the president's re-election strategy is failing. Despite a wave of voter suppression efforts—including slow mail service and new restrictions on late-arriving ballots—early voting continues at an epic pace with eighty million votes cast already. Joe Biden, the challenger, has a ten-point lead nationwide. Four days to go.

OCTOBER 30, 2020

	Cases	Deaths	Deaths/Million	Daily new
World:	45,892,274	1,193,240	153	573,616
US:	9,316,247	235,159	709	101,461

The US has reported over 100,000 new infections in one day. There have been half a million new positive infections in the US in the past week and 1,200 counties are now considered hot spots, surpassing all previous records in the nation.

Trump has been trying to make the case that "we are rounding the corner" and has obviously failed, so now he targets the doctors treating COVID and suggests they are inflating the infection numbers for profit. The healthcare community is outraged. While MAGA supporters flaunt public health safety protocols at Trump rallies, the doctors and nurses are feverishly working to save the lives he puts at risk for political gain.

The lieutenant governor in Idaho—our neighboring state—is trying to make a stand that is equally absurd. In a "declaration" video for an anti-lockdown group, she was recorded sitting in a pickup draped with giant American flags, holding a bible with a gun placed on top, and suggesting the pandemic is a hoax…that restrictions infringe on her freedom, and she will ignore them.

Her fellow Republican lawmakers also signed "the declaration" despite the record number of infections, overwhelmed hospitals, and rising deaths in the state. In some Idaho counties, when you need hospitalization for COVID they evacuate you to Seattle. There is no better example of false liberty than putting the lives of others at risk to preserve your own "rights."

On another front, Russian state sponsored hackers have attacked the electronic data systems of several hospitals, using ransomware ahead of the election. Cyber security experts have warned that the hackers have a list of four hundred hospitals to hit and so far, those targeted have all been in blue states—New York, Vermont and Oregon.

And adding to the chaos, two more Black men have been killed by police in the past week—one in Pennsylvania and one in Portland, Oregon—stirring up racial tensions and rioting by anarchists who once again seize opportunity.

It is difficult to describe the current level of stress in the country, but one leading journalist suggested this could be the last weekend of the nation as we know it. Late night comedians are hard-pressed to make jokes and admit that most of us are terrified; the president warns of "bedlam" in the streets.

Ninety million Americans have already voted with three days to go.

OCTOBER 31, 2020

Keith and I spent the day setting up Pandemic Porch, an outdoor space where we can entertain friends when it is cold. It took several hours to hang thick tarps across two exposed sides, string LED cafe lights, and position a propane heater under the high side of the slanted roof. There are rugs and lanterns and candles, and a bench seat filled with warm blankets. We hope this cozy porch allows us to have dinner with friends this fall and winter—outside.

The second wave is sweeping Europe with more than ten million infections to date. After flattening the curve last spring and living large this summer, the fall surge is now hitting hard and nearly a dozen countries have announced lockdowns starting tomorrow. France, Germany, Belgium, Ireland, Scotland, Wales, Greece and Austria will join Spain and Italy in closing bars, restaurants, theaters and gyms for a month. Most countries are trying to keep schools open, but the high hospitalization rate requires strict mitigation measures.

In the UK, leaders will also close public spaces starting Monday until December 2 due to a record number of infections, hospitalizations and deaths that exceed even the worst-case scenarios.

The US is now beyond every pandemic projection issued as a dire warning during the summer. Dr. Fauci finally had enough and spoke freely about the failure of this administration to control the pandemic and the danger of the misinformation Dr. Atlas is spreading. During an interview with *The Washington Post,* he said, "We're in for a whole lot of hurt. It's not a good situation," he said, referring to the current surge. "We're nearing 100,000 cases a day. All the stars are aligned in the wrong place as you go into the fall and winter season, with people congregating at home indoors. You could not possibly be positioned more poorly."

The Washington Post interview with Dr. Fauci was published the same day a Russian disinformation network aired an interviewed with

Dr. Atlas filmed at the White House during which he repeated all the herd immunity misinformation he has been feeding the president. He later apologized and said he had no idea the network was sponsored by Russians.

Dr Fauci wondered aloud why President Trump is listening to a radiologist with no experience instead of a team of infectious disease specialists who have advised every president for the past fifty years. Millions of sick and suffering Americans are wondering the same thing. Two days to go.

NOVEMBER 2, 2020

We are on the eve of a presidential election that is the most important in my lifetime. Nearly a hundred million Americans have voted early, and millions of return ballots are still in the mail. We may reach a new record in voter turnout—150 million or more.

There are thousands of court cases to either limit or expand the counting of ballots; voter intimidation tactics are making the rounds on social media. International observers expect to see armed militias at polling places, "trains" of Trump supporters clogging traffic, court interference as ballots are counted, premature victory announcements. Security officials are putting up a wall around the White House that cannot be climbed, and store owners in some cities are boarding up windows.

The challenger is clearly favored to win according to one renowned pollster. Yet those who are hoping for change are suffering PTSD from four years ago when the favored candidate won the popular vote by three million and yet lost the electoral college to Trump due to razor-thin margins in three states. Could it happen again?

The stakes could not be higher. We are in the middle of a pandemic and headed for a catastrophic rise during the coming winter. The economic damage is beyond imagination, with more than fifty percent of businesses at risk of failing. We see armed militias responding to racial tensions, and angry groups clash on American streets after every suspicious death of a Black citizen by a White cop… and there are many. The pain and suffering seem endless.

But instead of being paralyzed by fear the American voter is fighting back, answering the call to action, planning to vote, participating in democracy at historic levels. Whatever happens tomorrow, I am proud to be an American today.

NOVEMBER 3, 2020

Election Day

Nine am: Everything is up in the air, with some saying we may know the results tonight if Florida turns blue or if the opposition to President Trump is overwhelming or if a handful of red states flip in an election night surprise.

I am preparing snacks for a long night, making the guest room ready for my brother and his wife who are the only people currently in our COVID careful bubble, and chilling champagne just in case. Stay tuned!

Twelve pm: The polls were busy early but now there is a steady flow of voters waiting less than an hour in most cases. One elated attorney general said the election was "boring." With 102 million voters returning ballots early, in-person voting on election day is for those who were not willing to take any of the COVID careful options. I am reminded of Y2K fear, the widespread belief that every computer would be wiped clean when the century ended at midnight in the first minute of the year 2000…but it did not happen.

Twelve am (November 4): The returns are trickling in, and the race is close; results will take several days to confirm. The ten-point lead for Joe Biden disappeared under a wave of same-day voting by Trump supporters. The election was peaceful, and the streets were calm. There was no indication of meddling by other nations and no voter intimidation.

Despite millions of ballots still to be counted, President Trump just declared victory and suggested it was time to stop counting the votes. He threatened to take it to the Supreme Court, although no one can provide a reason. It is a tense night, and we steel our nerves with wine and poker and check the results at regular intervals; it's our first all-nighter in decades.

NOVEMBER 4, 2020

In the past few months, many of the president's supporters suggested that the pandemic would be over today because it was a hoax designed to hurt his re-election chances. So, it is ironic that the US had another record high for infections in the past 24 hours—over 108,000 people tested positive for the virus the day after the election. Considering how many thousands attended rallies in states with the highest cases during the past three weeks, the dark winter Dr. Fauci predicted is likely to come true.

Most of the election results reported today are favorable to Biden, who may beat the incumbent, which has happened only three times in the past one hundred years. Trump is losing in several battleground states and has filed lawsuits to end vote counting where he is currently ahead—Pennsylvania and Georgia—since he is facing an avalanche of mail-in votes that will not be in his favor.

On another front, there were rumors that hundreds of thousands of ballots are currently languishing at post offices and have not been delivered despite an order to deliver issued by a federal judge. The same judge ordered USPS to sweep post offices and search for those missing ballots prior to the election deadline of 8 pm yesterday but it was not done. The judge is not happy and has threatened to bring the Postmaster General—the Republican fundraiser appointed by the president last June—into the court to answer for the delay.

The presidential election is a nail-biter, and it looks like the Republicans will hold the Senate. Obviously, the pandemic failure was of no concern to voters in red states and win or lose, President Trump is not likely to ease our pain even though winter is coming.

November 5, 2020

Due to lawsuits and protests to "Stop the count" by Trump supporters, the count has been slowed. On the other side, there are people marching in several cities chanting "Count every vote." How could America come to this? Wear a mask.... don't wear a mask. Count the votes...don't count the votes.

People who would never think to stop a sporting event until the clock runs out are now insisting we stop counting thousands of mail-in votes because they are currently ahead. Unfortunately, President Trump, his family, and his lawyers have taken to conservative media and are shouting that the votes now being counted are fake votes, planted by Democrats to steal the election. And people believe it due to four years of brainwashing about voter fraud by the president.

However, despite commissions and court cases and non-profit groups who have looked and looked and looked again, no voter fraud of any import has been found. Fortunately, the men and women responsible for safe and fair voting are dedicated professionals and intend to count every vote regardless of political pressure.

New unemployment claims for the past week were 751,000.

November 6, 2020

This is the fourth day of counting votes in the election for the US president and Joe Biden is gaining ground. Again, President Trump's party has asked the Supreme Court to stop the count in Pennsylvania, but they refused. Most of the fringe lawsuits Trump has filed in the state courts have been thrown out as well.

The president continues to tweet about the "stolen election," and 37% of those tweets have been labeled as misinformation. His speech from the White House last night was so full of false accusations of fraud, several networks ended the broadcast two minutes in. Many have said it was the most dishonest speech of his entire presidency; his social media posts have been flagged as misinformation. Even his political supporters are asking for proof of fraud, but there is no proof. The votes are being counted like they always are...carefully.

The soon-to-be president-elect, Joe Biden, gave a speech tonight focusing on his priorities: the pandemic, the economy, climate change, and racial justice. President-elect Biden stressed unity for Americans and asked that we stay calm while the process of counting the votes concludes. He did not claim victory but was confident he would win.

The people of the United States have always enjoyed a peaceful transfer of power and the next two months should start with the proverbial handshake between opponents after a contest. But Trump says he will not concede or participate in the transfer of power if he loses. Many are prepared for even more chaos.

NOVEMBER 7, 2020

The American voters have rejected Donald Trump, who brought division, incompetence, indifference, racism, misogyny, narcissism, and xenophobia to the White House; the American people have chosen to pursue a more perfect union, to include and eventually unite the diversity that is the true character of our nation.

Amid a pandemic, 150 million have cast their vote—a record number—spending hours in line or driving miles to a drop box to ensure their vote was counted. They cast a vote for the first minority female vice president and the oldest man to reach the nation's highest office. "Democracy beats deep in the heart of America," Biden said after his win was announced.

People are flooding the streets to celebrate the end of the worst presidency in American history, as ranked by every historian on record. It is a jubilant celebration, with nearly everyone in face masks and some dispensing hand sanitizer to those around them. We have a bottle of champagne on ice to open when the president-elect speaks to the nation tonight.

Although Trump has promised not to concede and to bring even more lawsuits next week, his legacy will be cemented by what he does in the next few days and weeks. He becomes the tenth president to be rejected by voters after one term, and there has never been a one-term president who refused to concede.

Regardless of the missing concession, world leaders are congratulating the president-elect…with a big sigh of relief: "Welcome back, America," the mayor of Paris said with bells ringing in the background. The reputation of American democracy has been restored. People are in the streets around the world, celebrating with us.

Unfortunately, today we saw another record high for virus infections and there are nearly 250,000 Americans dead from the pandemic. The president-elect has promised to address the pandemic as a first order of business despite the losing president's refusal. A new virus task force is being assembled and will begin work before the inauguration due to an overwhelming necessity.

I will never forget this historic election. "Trust the people" I told my friend… and the people have spoken.

NOVEMBER 8, 2020

Trump refuses to concede and vows to "fight" to keep his base energized. Armed supporters have taken up their posts outside election centers where the count is ongoing. Despite zero evidence for Trump's claims of election fraud, Republican leaders remain silent because they believe that his base and his blessing is their only way to retain power. Cowards, all.

The transition has already begun. The president-elect will announce his new virus task force tomorrow, naming thirteen epidemiologists and scientists to lead us forward. It will be a tremendous relief to hear credible science from our nation's new leaders. As President-elect Biden said during his speech to the nation yesterday:

"We cannot repair the economy, restore our vitality or relish life's most precious moments—hugging a grandchild, birthdays, weddings, graduations, all the moments that matter most to us—until we get this virus under control," Biden said. "That plan will be built on a bedrock of science. It will be constructed out of compassion, empathy and concern. I will spare no effort—or commitment—to turn this pandemic around."

The US has recorded over 100,000 infections in the past 24 hours for the fifth day in a row…an indication of how much work has been left undone.

NOVEMBER 9, 2020

Today there is very good news and very bad news. The good news is that a vaccine developed by the Pfizer (and BioNTech in Germany) looks very promising with a 90% effective rate for developing antibodies and preventing virus infections. They will apply for emergency use authorization at the end of the month and have a limited supply available in late December if all goes well.

The Pfizer Phase 3 trial was aided by the fact that infections are rising so quickly in the US that test subjects were exposed at a much faster rate than expected. There are eleven vaccine candidates worldwide in Phase 3 trials and six that have been granted some provisional use. There is light at the end of this dark tunnel.

The bad news: Today is the sixth day in a row with over 100,000 infections in the US and there is concern that we can reach 200,000 per day by Christmas. Although the death rate is down between 1% and 2% due to better treatment options, the hospitals and morgues cannot handle all the sick and the dead. There are field hospitals going up—in winter—to handle the surge.

All fifty states are seeing an increase in positive tests and eighteen states have implemented additional lockdown restrictions. The city of Denver—where Michael, Kevin and Rachel live—has instituted a "Home by 10" order which means people must remain in their homes between 10 p.m. and 5 a.m., except for essential services—a curfew. The order prohibits all public and private gatherings between people from different households—except Thanksgiving Day.

We are headed into a very bleak winter with community spread of the virus so out of control that contract tracing is impossible; most people do not know how or where they contracted the virus. In just ten months we went from one case to ten million cases and might double the number again in two months; the president-elect may have no option but to shut down the country as his first official order of business after his inauguration on January 20.

NOVEMBER 10, 2020

Hospitalizations for COVID infections have reached a record high at nearly 62,000 and the worst is yet to come with the trend for infections up nearly 70%. Sickness and death will follow: Nearly 1,500 people died from the virus in the past 24 hours.

El Paso, Texas has the highest number of hospitalizations at 1,073 and has surpassed all surge capacity. They set up ten mobile morgues, a field hospital at the university, and added tents to the hospital parking lot to handle the surge. They are evacuating patients by helicopter to other Texas hospitals but with nearly 13,000 new cases in the past 24 hours, Texas is in trouble. They have the distinction of being the first state to report over one million cases in ten months.

Since the entire nation is a hot spot, there is no possibility of additional medical personnel traveling to places hardest hit; most states are either near or at capacity and there are few reserves. Asymptomatic but virus positive medical personnel are being called in from quarantine to treat the surge in COVID patients. No one knows what effect more exposure might have on asymptomatic status.

The federal response is nonexistent; Trump is too busy filing frivolous lawsuits and tweeting about voter fraud to consider the pain and suffering of Americans. He refuses to concede or allow the peaceful transition of power. The world watches as democracy is infected by his hunger for power.

NOVEMBER 11, 2020

There are two Senate seats in Georgia that are headed to a runoff due to a state law that requires winners to receive more than 50% of the vote; both seats are still open and will be decided on January 5. With the Senate now at 48/50, two Democratic wins in Georgia could flip the Senate to the president-elect's party. The state is already looking blue…but just barely.

For this reason, Republican leaders have backed President Trump's claim that the election was stolen even though the public has already accepted the result. The president continues to rally his MAGA base (some say for money) with claims of a stolen election. Republicans need to win the two Georgia seats to retain control of the Senate, so they repeat the stolen election lies. It is surreal to watch so many career politicians spend so much political capital trying to protect the ego of a losing president at the expense of the nation.

The 2020 lame duck session is lamer than ever since the transition plans of the winning administration are delayed by a losing administration that is trying to execute a coup while a pandemic rages. It is estimated that if nothing more is done to control the spread, the US will have 300,000 cases a day before the inauguration on January 20…an object lesson in nearly exponential growth.

What we cannot grow exponentially are hospital beds and PPE, nurses and doctors, morgues and crematoriums. We were repeatedly warned about the winter wave, and it is descending upon us. There have never been enough tests, and nearly half the country refuses to wear a mask for political reasons. One essential player in this dark political tragedy that is not a lame duck is the virus; the virus is thriving.

NOVEMBER 12, 2020

The unemployment figures were released for last week with 709,000 new claims filed for regular unemployment and 248,000 filed for those not usually covered by state plans. There are currently 6.8 million receiving benefits through the states, with an unemployment rate of around 7%.

This rate does not include all the working mothers who have given up jobs to care for their children at home. Women are still more likely than men to keep the home fires burning and to educate the children. It is an especially stressful time for one parent households. I cannot imagine how one person can be responsible for raising and educating children and still have the resources needed to provide a home.

It will get worse. At the end of the year, many of the benefits of the stimulus extension will expire. This will mean foreclosure for those who have not been able to pay rent or mortgages, and a reduction in unemployment funds for those who lost jobs early in the pandemic.

With the catastrophic rise in infection rates, new shutdowns are inevitable. Those who have barely hung on will lose their grip and join the millions of other Americans who do not know how they will support their family in the coming months. Since the president is now ignoring the pandemic and the Senate has no incentive to provide support, we are on our own until January 20.

NOVEMBER 13, 2020

Well, the North Dakota governor has finally cried "UNCLE" and ordered a mask mandate and limits on gatherings for the first time.

He also required asymptomatic nurses to return to work on COVID floors, which was only allowed after a crisis declaration.

The South Dakota governor is still holding out, priding herself on having no restrictions in the state after hosting the biggest super-spreader events in the country including the Fourth of July extravaganza with the president at Mount Rushmore, the annual state fair, and the Sturgis motorcycle rally in August—an action-packed summer.

And now the Dakotas have the highest infection rate per capita in the world, at 70,000 cases per million for the South and 80,000 for the North. "I have no intention of enforcing mandates with federal money," the South Dakota governor said in response to Biden's warning that mask mandates were needed. She cited personal freedom, of course, and considers herself a patriot.

Positive tests results for COVID doubled in two weeks, from 85,000 on Halloween to 183,000 today. Since hospitalizations and deaths lag by two weeks on average, the current over-capacity surge at hospitals is only half of what it will be when a record-breaking number of people with current infections seek care for their life-threatening illness.

In the past seven days, the US has seen a daily average of 140,000 new positive cases. There is no place on the planet close to our daily infection rate.... the next highest yesterday was India with 45,000.

And let this sink in: We had 183,000 new positive cases today.

There were partial lockdowns announced in Oregon and New Mexico, concerns about keeping public schools open in New York, and nationwide questions about sending college students home for Thanksgiving. We need to shut down for at least four weeks to manage this surge, but the soon-to-be ex-president Trump spoke from the Rose Garden and said there will be no national lockdown. Absolutely not.

Part Three: Insurrection

November 15-January 20, 2021

November 15, 2020

	Cases	Deaths	Deaths/Million	Daily new
World:	54,312,999	1,317,414	169	575,843
US:	11,226,218	251,2256	757	157,253

EMERGENCY ROOM NURSE IN SOUTH DAKOTA:

I have a night off from the hospital. As I'm on my couch with my dog I can't help but think of the COVID patients the last few days. The ones that stick out are those who still don't believe the virus is real. The ones who scream at you for a magic medicine and that Joe Biden is going to ruin the USA. All the while gasping for breath on 100% Vapotherm. They tell you there must be another reason they are sick. They call you names and ask why you have to wear all that "stuff" because they don't have COVID because it's not real.

* * *

Of all the dystopian novels I have read over the past fifty years, none has felt as dark as the composite scene described above by an

ICU nurse in South Dakota—nor as true. The current surge is an unfolding of a knowing…and we have no collective will to stop it.

Thousands of President Trump's far-right supporters, marshaled by Fox News, gathered on Freedom Plaza to protest "the stolen election." What they did not wear—a mask—was as telling as the red, white, and blue symbols of patriotism they did wear. Trump thanked these misinformed and angry White nationalists via Twitter and waved from the limo on his way to play golf. Some of these folks will be part of the growing surge that will once again overwhelm the country in another few weeks, joining those who gather with friends and family for Thanksgiving in eleven days.

Our annual feast has been cancelled this year. Hannah will drive to Colorado for Thanksgiving, then quarantine with Michael and Kevin and Rachel before they drive here in mid-December. They have never missed a Christmas at home. My brother and his wife will join us for a small turkey dinner on Thanksgiving Day. It is too cold for a long afternoon on Pandemic Porch and too risky to host friends indoors.

NOVEMBER 16, 2020

Infections in Sweden have doubled in the past two weeks; the herd immunity failure is even more apparent now that cold weather has forced the public indoors. At a news conference today, the Prime Minister announced restrictions that will become the "new norm" for this country going forward: "Don't go to the gym. Don't go to the library. Don't have dinners. Don't have parties. Cancel," he said.

The US has recorded one million new infections in the past six days with rates rising in forty-eight states. New closures are announced hourly which now include Illinois, Pennsylvania, Michigan, Washington, New Jersey, California and Washington, in addition to the partial shutdown in Oregon starting tomorrow. Many Republican governors are issuing mask mandates for the first time.

In response to the Michigan closures, Dr. Atlas—the discredited radiologist informing the current president—tweeted: "The only way this stops is if people rise up. You get what you accept." He has since realized that his tweet might incite (more) violence in Michigan where a plot to kidnap Governor Gretchen Whitmer was recently discovered, and he retracted his statement. The lunatics are running the asylum.

Trump still refuses to concede his election loss and will not release the information President-elect Biden needs to begin planning a pandemic response. Not only does Trump refuse to address this once-in-a-century crisis, but he is also holding critical pandemic information hostage. Every lost day means less testing, fewer coordinated mitigation efforts, no pre-planning for vaccine distribution… and more unnecessary death.

Republican senators remain silent regarding the election loss; every single one refused to be interviewed by the news media this weekend. The lack of backbone among these leaders is stunning.

The nation is in the middle of an unmitigated health disaster and millions of healthcare workers are at the end of their rope. Keith is concerned about an increase in suicide among physicians, which means there will be more deaths to lay at the feet of this incompetent president.

NOVEMBER 17, 2020

While most of us are not compelled to rock the boat, a person with an emotional disorder does so to feel secure and ends up making everyone in the boat seasick…rocking, rocking, rocking. See what I can do? Are you watching me? I'm the greatest, right?

The entire world is watching this man-child throw a tantrum, rocking a boat that has been breached and is taking on water; a boat that will soon sink.

It is a dangerous time for the nation—for any nation—when a disturbed man desperately grips the helm, clinging to power. We hope our ship of state is sound.

NOVEMBER 18, 2020

The world has received good news about vaccine development in the past two weeks. Pfizer has data showing their vaccine is more than 90% effective and is seeking FDA approval for emergency use. Moderna has also announced development of a vaccine with 95% effectiveness and will be seeking approval for emergency use. One of the most successful endeavors of the current administration is Operation Warp Speed, an "all-hands-on-deck" strategy for rapid vaccine development, and the production of every element needed for the actual vaccine.

There is hope that some healthcare workers can receive the first dose next month. Discussions regarding how to distribute the vaccine are ongoing due to the complexity of shipping and storing and deciding who should be first. These decisions must consider employment and age and race if the distribution is to be fair and effective.

There are other vaccine options currently in phase three trials that are moving along rapidly due to the surge in virus cases and the data that follows. Most people will be able to receive a vaccine to protect them from COVID in 2021, but all of us will need strong assurances that the vaccine is safe.

NOVEMBER 19, 2020

In a normal year, I would be finalizing plans with the twenty-plus people who would be gathering around our fourteen-foot table for Thanksgiving dinner and making room for a 25-pound turkey in the fridge, but not this year. I stuffed all my inclinations to host as deep as possible...so deep we may never have twenty people at the table again despite thirty years of being the go-to host for holiday gatherings.

In a normal year, I would be canvassing family about Christmas and questioning friends about their plans. "Come for Christmas!"

is usually how those conversations end but not this year. This year I quietly implement plans to help my three adult children celebrate Christmas in Denver in case one of them tests positive in the next few weeks.

We are approaching 200,000 cases per day as predicted and 2,000 people died of COVID yesterday. Hospitals are already full of the sick and the morgues are filling up. Some say Trump is traumatized by his election loss and unable to think about anything else. He is laser focused on overturning the election and only mentions the pandemic when he takes credit for Operation Warp Speed, which he deserves.

The American Automobile Association (AAA) estimates that fifty million people are planning to travel for Thanksgiving; 40% will celebrate with more than ten people. Warnings from the CDC to stay home are falling on deaf ears. The virus deniers—and those with pandemic fatigue—are convinced the benefits outweigh the risks.

State unemployment claims increased by 743,000 last week. The Pandemic Emergency Unemployment Insurance (PEUI) will end on December 26 unless Congress passes another spending stimulus bill. If not, twelve million workers will permanently lose the Federal insurance that temporarily extended state benefits.

NOVEMBER 20, 2020

A woman in South Dakota gave an interview for a NYT reporter and is quoted saying "Those who wear masks are losing their soul and America is next!" South Dakota is approaching a 50% positive test rate—the highest in the nation—but the virus denier quoted above is planning to host Thanksgiving dinner for twenty people as usual… and proud of it.

The South Dakota governor has refused to consider anything that might infringe on "liberty" and people agree. On any given Friday night there are football games, dances, weddings, and the restaurants are full. The unemployment rate is fifty percent lower than the rest of the nation while the infection rate is fifty percent higher, an interesting juxtaposition.

South Dakota is conducting an experiment in herd immunity like Sweden, a nation that survived the early wave without closing but the elderly paid a high price. Sweden was still forced to shut down during the oncoming winter wave. The virus took out the easy targets first and then came back when the weather crowded people indoors. Now the virus finds all the places where people are willfully unprotected and takes advantage of their stubborn independence.

America is a country where stubborn independence can make people sick. There is no place in the world where personal freedom is more celebrated than in the land of the red, white, and blue; no place where the virus has found such an inviting home. And once again we see that personal freedom requires personal responsibility; without responsibility there is no freedom.

NOVEMBER 21, 2020

Italy was the first western nation to record deaths from COVID, the first country to completely close, and one of the last to re-open due to the severity of the outbreak in early March. After a relatively controlled summer, Italy is again in the news with 10,000 deaths last month—two times the per capita rate in the US. Italians have a severe case of pandemic fatigue, so this new surge is no longer causing a national panic, just hundreds of deaths…seven hundred today.

Nearly one million people in the United States traveled on a plane yesterday—the most since March—despite the CDC and the rest of the nation's epidemiologists begging us to stay home, warning us that Thanksgiving feasts will lead to Christmas funerals, that the virus will join the holiday table and send the beloved back home with a deadly disease. Asymptomatic spread is still responsible for fifty percent of new cases.

Michael and Rachel and Kevin are in quarantine after the chef at Lost City Coffee tested positive. All three are scheduled for a COVID test as a precaution. Colorado and Oregon are both reaching record-high positive rates and in the beginning stages of a second shutdown.

NOVEMBER 22, 2020

From recent experience I know how easy it is to let down your guard, to completely ignore the implications of a particular plan until it is too late. I scheduled an appointment with a cable technician to upgrade our system without considering that I also had plans for games and lunch with my brother and his wife during the same time on Saturday. The conflict did not dawn on me until both were on their way.

I checked the safety protocols for the cable company, reviewed the risk with Keith, and quickly checked in with my brother but none of us were overly concerned. We would keep the windows open, and the technician would be masked.

All went well until the end of the installation. We were too close when he asked for signatures, when he explained the new system, when we asked questions about his recent move to the county, about his family. We were polite as we engaged in this risky behavior—speaking with a stranger unmasked indoors, with too little distance between us. The fourteen-day countdown begins.

NOVEMBER 24, 2020

2,194 deaths from COVID in 24 hours

With a record 85,000 ICU patients, hospitals have reached capacity and are also seriously challenged by a shortage of nurses.

The US death rate from COVID dropped from an average of 5.5% (March to June) to a steady 1.7% since July due to more testing and medical capacity and better treatment—including monoclonal antibodies. But with too few ICU beds and experienced nurses and a million new infections each week, deaths will rise along with our nation's status as the leader of pandemic failures. We are truly exceptional.

Our failure is partly due to the ongoing success of the virus to reinvent itself. Before jumping continents, the virus mutated and the strain that reached the East and West coasts of the US was much more contagious than the early strain in Europe. Epidemiologists labeled the new variant 614G and then traced the strain from Italy to the Americas over the spring. In January and February only 5% of the confirmed cases in the US had the variant, but by March it was 72%; in June, 98% of virus infections in the US were caused by the much more contagious 614G strain.

The pandemic we are experiencing in most of the western world is the result of a clever biological threat—with an innate ability to adapt—making war upon a host population unwilling to raise a defense. To thwart the enemy, we would need to isolate for another month and then use masks and physical distance to limit the risk, but the virus adapts faster than human nature so we will continue to suffer and die until science can save us.

NOVEMBER 25, 2020

2,304 deaths from COVID in 24 hours

The millions upon millions of Americans who are traveling for Thanksgiving are playing Russian Roulette with their friends and families while the world watches in dumbfounded disbelief. Most of Europe is still in lockdown with a goal of slowly lifting restrictions by Christmas. Americans will face the music for their reckless Thanksgiving three weeks from now. Experts predict the death rate will double.

Hannah finished her finals and hitched a ride with a friend to Denver. She reassures us they have both been isolating in their respective apartments, had negative COVID tests before they left, and will take every precaution during the eighteen-hour drive. Michael and Rachel and Kevin all tested negative as well. What else can be done? I am thankful they are isolating together.

New unemployment claims for last week were released a day early and 828,000 were filed, which is an increase of 78,000 over last week. The lines at food banks stretch for miles in the nation's urban areas. There is no additional help coming from our government.

NOVEMBER 27, 2020

Here is a recap of the first two waves of the 2020 pandemic: The first wave of the "new virus" in the US started in the East and West coastal cities simultaneously due to travelers entering through the major airports in Seattle, New York and Los Angeles starting in February. In New York specifically, the outbreak was so bad that field hospitals were set up in Central Park and thousands of unidentified COVID dead were buried on Hart Island.

The New York governor pleaded for help and states responded with healthcare workers and PPE and ventilators. Medical personnel were considered heroes and were celebrated with flowers and pizza and a chorus of applause each night from street corners and balconies. The country went into lockdown to reserve hospital capacity but reopened two months later due to economic concerns.

The second wave moved through the Deep South starting mid-August, but the Republican governors in those states did not require masks and were open for business as usual, which allowed the virus to spread through the Midwest. There were no coordinated mitigation efforts, but treatment improved and so did the death rate. Praise for the medical community was replaced by suspicion that the pandemic was being used as a political tool to benefit Democrats; public health officials received death threats for proposals based on science and physicians were accused of profiteering.

In the first two waves the highest number of hospitalizations recorded for the nation was 60,000 a day, which stressed the system. There were lockdowns in the first wave and medical evacuations from rural to urban hospitals in the second.

And now we have the third wave. Today it was reported that there are 90,000 severe COVID patients in the hospital—an increase of 40% in two weeks—with more than a million new infections every week and rising. And when the infection rate rises, an increase in hospitalization follows; when the hospitalization rate rises, an increase in death follows.

The hospitals are overwhelmed, and experts now predict that the death rate in the US will double in the next few weeks due to millions of new infections reported this fall… just in time for Christmas.

NOVEMBER 28, 2020

Breaking News: A vaccine to prevent the virus is airborne. Tens of millions of Pfizer COVID-19 vaccine vials are in the air, flying to Chicago onboard a United plane as part of distribution pre-placement in advance of FDA approval scheduled for December 10. Once the expected approval is granted, a network of commercial jetliners will distribute vaccine to all fifty states. The Moderna vaccine is expecting FDA approval on December 19 with distribution to quickly follow.

It took just sixty-three days from receipt of the virus genome sequence to development of a vaccine using messenger RNA and testing on human subjects, which is a record for vaccine development and a first for mRNA technology—a real medical breakthrough decades in the making.

Not only did we find a vaccine for COVID in record time, but we also found a way to use genetic strands to communicate new instructions to diseased cells, a new technology that has been in development for twenty years and has implications for future viruses and a wide range of other medical applications.

Each state must decide the priority for access to the vaccine starting with healthcare providers and the elderly. Distribution will be the next challenge, since the vaccine must be held below -94 degrees in specially-designed boxes that can only be opened twice a day. Each box can hold up to five-thousand doses that must be used within five days once opened.

Full inoculation will require two doses per person a few weeks apart, so rural communities will be challenged to distribute a full box of vaccine in a five-day period without wasting doses. But given the quality of the science to date, I have every confidence that these problems will be solved.

Currently we are told that mass inoculation will require another four to six months in the US. At last, we see a faint light at the end of the tunnel.

NOVEMBER 30, 2020

	CASES	DEATHS	DEATHS/MILLION	DAILY NEW
WORLD:	63,596,281	1,473,549	189	499,541
US:	13,920,038	274,332	827	161,736

President Trump has lost every lawsuit he filed alleging election fraud—nearly forty suits in battleground states—and still he tweets about the "stolen" election and refuses to concede.

He is focused on destruction. Destruction of the peaceful transition of American power; of the career civilian service corps; of our relationships with allies and the treaties he has yet to shred; of the humane rules the government must follow to execute prisoners. He and his DOJ favor the firing squad and hope to change the rules so they can shoot as many as possible before the inauguration on January 20—even though there has never been a federal execution during a lame-duck session. He plays golf and rants "I won!" like a mad king and ponders how many presidential pardons to sell. It seems that everything in America is for sale.

Americans are sick and dying from the pandemic in record numbers as anticipated by public health officials as winter arrives. What was not anticipated is that we would face the worst wave without any preparation by the federal government or financial help for the states. Again, hospitals do not have enough protective gear or personnel or beds; and still, the public has too little testing to know if it is safe to travel for the holidays...so they travel anyway.

A catastrophe is upon us once again, a greater catastrophe than we experienced in the first two waves; soon-to-be the greatest public health failure in American history, and it could have been prevented.

DECEMBER 1, 2020

2,614 US deaths in 24 hours

Dr. Atlas, who tried to convince the president to adopt a herd-immunity strategy, publicly congratulated himself on his success and then resigned. The rest of the virus task force is breathing a sigh of relief. With one death from COVID every minute in the US, success is hardly the word to describe our response as a nation.

In Oregon we reached 25,000 cases in six months, 50,000 cases in another two months, and a high of 75,000 cases three weeks later; most of the state is in the red zone except where we live, which has the lowest risk. We do not trust the reporting, however, since we have too few tests at the end of the road.

In Colorado, the governor and his partner have both tested positive and are in quarantine—along with governors of six other states. The mayor of Denver created a political firestorm when he tweeted that everyone should stay home on Thanksgiving...just before boarding a plane to Mississippi to celebrate the holiday with his family. Like most states, Colorado had a brutal November, going from 2,000 to an average of 5,000 new infections every day; one in every forty-one residents is thought to be contagious.

Our children in Denver are developing a Christmas travel protocol and asking for our approval. We will take some risk but not much with vaccines just a few months away. The four of them will quarantine together for eight days—no friends, just delivery food—with a test midweek before they travel. They will share a room on the outskirts of Salt Lake City mid-trip and arrive here on the tenth day—December 21. They have masks and sanitizer and disinfectant wipes.

DECEMBER 2, 2020

2,833 deaths in 24 hours
100,300 currently hospitalized with COVID

We have surpassed 100,000 hospitalizations for COVID even before the Thanksgiving toll becomes apparent and more than two thousand are dying each day. Dr. Redfield, director of the CDC, warned that the next three months will be the most difficult months in US public health history. He predicts we will reach a death toll of over 450,000 Americans by February.

They have recruited prisoners to help move bodies to mobile morgues in El Paso and to set up a makeshift COVID ward for two hundred in a parking lot in Reno. When the lame-duck president saw a picture of this heroic effort he tweeted that this was an obvious sign that the pandemic was a hoax. Really?

Even the Facebook founder is appalled at the damaging misinformation already circulating regarding the safety of vaccines and promised to remove all posts with false vaccine claims from the platform. Three past US presidents have volunteered to take the vaccine in front of the cameras to counter the damage being done by tweets and conspiracy blogs.

The secretary of state has invited nine hundred people to his holiday parties and the White House is hosting nearly two dozen events with masks advised but not provided—the final super-spreader events before the virus deniers leave the White House.

DECEMBER 3, 2020

2,918 COVID deaths in 24 hours

The governor of California announced he was "pulling an emergency break" today with a regional say-at-home order for each of five specified regions with less than 15% ICU capacity remaining. The order gives each region 24 hours to gain additional ICU capacity or immediately shut down for three weeks. Under the stay-at-home order, retail stores will be open with a maximum at 20% capacity, while bars, wineries, personal-service businesses, hair salons and barbershops will be closed.

President-elect Biden has put together his virus task force which includes Dr. Fauci in the top position. They will ask everyone in the nation to wear masks for the first one hundred days of the new administration to slow the winter surge, but there is little optimism that this request will be followed.

Pfizer announced a fifty percent reduction in the number of vaccines they can produce this year, from a hundred million down to fifty million doses due to problems with raw materials in the supply chain not meeting quality standards. Two steps forward and one step back.

DECEMBER 4, 2020

2,718 COVID deaths in 24 hours

We have gained invaluable knowledge about the pandemic over the past nine months:

We know that homes for the elderly are responsible for many deaths from the virus; we know that underlying health conditions—diabetes, hypertension, obesity—affect forty-five percent of the population and provide the next best killing field. We know that poverty and a concentration of minimum-wage workers guarantees that the working poor in minority neighborhoods suffer disproportionately;

we know that social and economic factors put people at risk, not the color of their skin.

We know that the same people who are most susceptible to illness and death from the virus are also more likely to suffer economic consequences in each successive wave of infection. People employed in the service industry—who were forced to close due to lockdowns—are low-wage employees who have limited access to unemployment insurance...or health insurance.

We know that employment insurance is designed as a narrow bridge between jobs and provides a fraction of replacement income for the unemployed; we know that when the emergency pandemic benefits issued last April end, thirteen million people without jobs will receive no income the next month even though the worst wave of the pandemic and the greatest public health crisis in US history is upon us.

We also know that in a crisis, the rich get richer, and the poor get poorer because the pyramid of inequality created by unregulated capitalism forces human suffering downhill; in a pandemic, an impossibly heavy weight of suffering descends upon the poor.

DECEMBER 5, 2020

I stumbled upon a series in the Washington Post titled "Voices from the Pandemic" by Eli Saslow who records and publishes the oral histories of those effected by COVID. He tells the story of a 67-year-old nursing home patient recovering from an accident who recounts the sound of rising infections moving from room to room...toward him. And a 78-year-old physician who is still practicing in a rural South Dakota clinic because fifty-percent of his patients are testing positive for the virus. And a Jamaican woman who passed the virus to her mother in a moment of weakness and then listened from a distance while her mother died in the bedroom upstairs.

These stories personalize the numbers and show the heartbreaking consequences of the pandemic as it ravages our country. Imagine the 290,000 stories of unnecessary deaths from COVID in the past nine months; imagine someone dying from the virus every forty seconds in this country; imagine it is someone you love.

DECEMBER 7, 2020

Eighty-five percent of California is under stay-at-home orders through December 28 because the ICU capacity is below fifteen percent as predicted. This means there are no private gatherings of any size, no non-essential businesses open for the holiday, no hotel rooms for out-of-state travelers unless they are essential AND can quarantine for fourteen days. They have asked the public to cancel holiday travel to California.

We have officially surpassed the death rate reached during the first wave in April, and we passed the daily infection record long ago. Hospitalizations have reached 101,000 and are holding only because there is little capacity left; the rate cannot go higher without erecting field hospitals in parking lots and parks. The Thanksgiving surge will begin soon…. just as people start traveling for Christmas. Dr. Fauci predicts an explosion of infection and death in mid-January, which seems likely since it took just five days to add another million infections last week.

Also predicted is an explosion in homelessness due to huge bills coming due for twelve million unemployed who owe nearly $6,000 each in back rent and thousands for unpaid utilities. There were only 245,000 jobs added in the entire month of November, half of what was expected. One in five restaurants have closed permanently and those jobs are lost for good; it is predicted that 10,000 more could close next week.

Congress has one week to avoid a catastrophe by passing another stimulus bill, but the odds are not good. There is a bi-partisan bill on the table, but the Senate Majority leader Mitch McConnell is pushing back, and Trump is still busy trying to overturn the election.

We also learned that the Trump administration failed to contract for additional Pfizer vaccines when offered five hundred million doses this summer, so they were sold to Britain and Europe; Britain started mass inoculations today. After the first one hundred million doses are distributed in the US to healthcare workers next month, it may be June before we see more doses, according to Pfizer.

DECEMBER 8, 2020

2,949 COVID deaths in 24 hours

I was struck by the timelessness of this quote from Sitting Bull (1830-1890) when his people were threatened and starving: "*The white man knows how to make everything, but he does not know how to distribute it.*" Sitting Bull often spoke about inequality, saying that the difference between the White man and the Red man is that the White man wants to keep everything and the Red man wants to give it away.

And this even earlier analysis from a Scottish historian, Sir Alex Fraser Tyler (1742-1813), also speaks to me:

The average age of the world's greatest civilizations has been two hundred years. These nations have progressed through this sequence:

From bondage to spiritual faith;
from spiritual faith to great courage;
from courage to liberty;
from liberty to abundance;
from abundance to selfishness;
from selfishness to complacency;
from complacency to apathy;
from apathy to dependence;
from dependency back again into bondage.

So, explain again how personal liberty is more important than the neighbor's health? How the virus is just a little flu and if we get it, we get it. What to do when we can't breathe and all the hospital beds are full? How to feed our families with an economy in ruins?

Tell me how a denial of science is not bondage.

DECEMBER 9, 2020

3,243 COVID deaths in 24 hours, another record

Dr. Fauci turns eighty on Christmas Eve but will not be spending his birthday or the holiday with his three daughters who all live in different cities. "We will miss being together for the holiday for the first time in thirty years," he said.

In contrast, the White House is in the middle of an active season of holiday parties with hundreds of guests who are photographed at "the people's house" without masks. Not a day goes by without hearing that some elected politician is in quarantine at home or in the hospital with COVID—a public servant receiving exceptional treatment and sick leave wages. There are too few public servants with the discipline to follow public health guidelines and too many who are "caught" breaking the rules and forced to apologize to their supporters. We are not "all in this together" no matter how often we hear it said.

Most of us are making life-and-death decisions daily. With evolving public health guidelines—on how much distance to keep, how easily COVID spreads indoors, how long a mask will protect—the most normal activity requires careful planning.

Yesterday Keith and I went to La Grande to activate a spare phone, sign papers for public health, and buy holiday supplies. We made five stops in 75 minutes which was in keeping with our rule to mask up and spend less than fifteen minutes at any indoor location. Our efficiency surprised us, and so did the kindness we were shown everywhere we went. We pondered whether it was our silver hair that stimulated such tender care, but it was greatly appreciated.

Our children text daily now, wondering what we think about their quarantine plan, which starts tomorrow. In quarantine, they will see only each other, visit no public (or even private) locations, and wear masks when walking outdoors. They have factored in a delay for test results and plan to drive sixteen hours in shifts to avoid the hotel; they will arrive here from Denver as a single quarantined household, and that means we can hug each other...if we also stay "safe."

DECEMBER 10, 2020

3,098 COVID deaths in 24 hours
107,258 people hospitalized with COVID
1.4 million new claims for unemployment last week

Although it has been forty days since Trump lost the election and all states have certified the results—despite fifty-five failed lawsuits seeking to stop the process including one summarily rejected by the Supreme Court last week—the losing president and his supporters are still trying to overturn the election.

The Texas Republican AG filed a second suit in the Supreme Court, claiming four states—Wisconsin, Pennsylvania, Michigan, and Georgia—suffered "unconstitutional irregularities" and that the results should be overturned. A brief supporting the case was signed by 106 members of the United States Congress and seventeen State Attorneys General—all Republicans—despite a complete lack of evidence.

Election officials in those four states have been victims of death threats and drive-by caravans of the president's supporters circling their neighborhoods and honking horns. Armed gangs gathered outside several Michigan homes with the intention of intimidating the ones who count the votes.

This alarming effort to subvert democracy has two goals: The first is to raise funds for the president's political future and the second is to provide insurance for incumbents. The Republicans who signed the loyalty pledge fear the president will retain enough power to mount primary challenges in 2022 against any Republican who does not support his coup attempt, so they go along.

Trump still claims, "I won!" at the super-spreader holiday parties being held at the White House, and he is still fundraising with over $250 million received since November 3rd for his "Stop the Steal!" campaign—money he desperately needs due to a debt of nearly half a billion dollars to mysterious and still unknown lenders listed on his most recent tax returns.

Because he does nothing to contain the pandemic and speaks only of the "stolen election," the damage of his failed presidency continues on two fronts: a catastrophic and uncontrolled public health crisis and a deliberate degradation of democracy. Well, there are three fronts if you count permanent damage to the integrity of the Republican party.

DECEMBER 11, 2020

3,031 COVID deaths in 24 hours

Two big announcements were made tonight: The Supreme Court refused to hear the Texas lawsuit, and the FDA approved the Pfizer vaccine for emergency use.

First the lawsuit. An additional twenty members of Congress and one more State Attorneys General (226/18 total) signed the supporting brief at the last minute—just a few hours before the Supreme Court issued the following statement: "*Texas has not demonstrated a judicially cognizable interest in the manner in which another State conducts its elections.*"

The vote was unanimous, the political fallout immediate. Terms like slander and sedition and treason are being bantered about. And yet, this humiliation is still not enough to stop Trump's cult of White male supremacy. The Texas Republican party is now talking about secession and evangelical supporters are headed to DC with Ram's horns to bring down the walls of Jericho—aptly called "the Jericho

March." It is important to keep in mind that Joe Biden won by over seven million votes. But some Republicans still claim that there were dead people voting despite a lack of proof. Maybe they can see dead people.

And finally, on Sunday the vaccine will begin shipping to all fifty states. Initially, just fifty million people will have access to the Pfizer vaccine—mainly healthcare workers and nursing home residents—but it looks like the Moderna vaccine will follow a week or two later. The effort to vaccinate a nation of 335 million is a heroic undertaking requiring airplanes and freezer trucks and pallets of vials, swabs and syringes, special onsite freezers, and a dozen other details that must be worked out. We are told it will take six months before everyone who is willing can be vaccinated.

Today over 246,000 people tested positive for the virus and in another three weeks thousands of them will be dead…too late to be saved by a new vaccine.

DECEMBER 12, 2020

2,307 COVID deaths in 24 hours
109,331 people in the hospital with COVID

There are several thousand marchers descending on D.C. and a few state capitals in "Stop the Steal" events today. The protests are in advance of the meeting of each state's Electoral College on Monday to cast electoral votes for the next president. The current president tweeted his support for the march and then drove by in his motorcade to signal thumbs up on his way to play more golf. Due to an alternative media that fuels a constant stream of misinformation, most of his supporters believe the myth of a stolen election despite a complete lack of evidence.

Trump hopes to control the Republican party after he leaves the White House on January 20, so the myth serves him well as do his hints of a 2024 presidential run. It remains to be seen how much power he retains after losing the presidency—especially when the lawsuits start stacking up.

DECEMBER 15, 2020

	Cases	Deaths	Deaths/Million	Daily new
World:	73,799,965	1,640,905	210.5	595,894
US:	17,145,459	311,093	937	201,552

The only thing missing from photos and videos of the Proud Boys marching around the nation's capital, screaming about a fictional stolen election and vandalizing Black churches, were the swastikas. They roamed the streets and looked for someone to fight. Remember when Trump was asked if he would denounce White supremacy during the September debate and his response was to tell the Proud Boys to "Stand back and stand by?" This weekend, four people were knifed and one was shot.

Keith and I spent Sunday afternoon delivering Christmas boxes with treats and candles to our friends, a family tradition. I was struck by the lack of decorations at most houses and the timid porch greetings. Like us, our friends have grown accustomed to isolation and answer the door with hope that the human being on the other side is COVID free; some answered in masks.

DECEMBER 16, 2020

3,538 COVID deaths in 24 hours
113,000 people in the hospital with COVID

Hospitals across the country are receiving their first box of COVID vaccine and first responders across the country have been photographed as they take the shot, some in tears.

At the same time, we shatter every record for infections, hospitalizations, and deaths daily. In southern California, they have 0%

ICU capacity and are forced to treat COVID patients in hallways and basements and parking lots.

Every five days one million more Americans test positive for the virus and every single day this week more than 3,000 have died. We are only halfway through December, but it is already the deadliest December in one hundred years—since the 1918 pandemic.

Think about this: There have been more COVID deaths in a day this December than during any day in any American war since 1862; more deaths than Normandy on D-Day when a record 2,500 US soldiers were killed; more deaths than on September 11, 2001, when 2,977 civilians died in a terrorist attack; more deaths every single day from an uncontrolled pandemic.

Eventually, we will win the COVID war if enough people receive the vaccine to produce herd immunity but every day until then we could lose thousands of our beloved soldiers.

DECEMBER 17, 2020

3,387 COVID deaths in 24 hours
114,237 people in hospitals with COVID

The king of Sweden apologized to the country in his Christmas address this year, saying, "I think we have failed. We have a large number who have died and that is terrible." When asked if he was concerned about catching the virus, he added, "Lately it has felt more obvious, it has crept closer and closer. That's not what you want."

Everyone knows how he feels about the virus closing in. Entire nations including this one have become hotspots. Ignoring the virus, making friends with the disease and allowing it to run freely in your country—in your house—has given it a stronger position from which to attack our every weakness.

Herd immunity can only be accomplished with a vaccine, as we have been told many times, and yet, by default, our government adopted the do-nothing strategy and let thousands die horrible and lonely deaths. Sweden's health minister let down his country; America's lame-duck president and his herd-immunity advisor let down ours.

Keith and I are another step closer to spending Christmas with our children. They are ten days into their quarantine and all tested negative for the virus this week. We feel a little guilty about our good fortune. Tens of millions of adult children do not have the luxury of working from home, of ordering groceries to be delivered, of driving home together as one unit. This year there are very few who casually ask if the children will be home for Christmas. For most, the answer is usually "not this year."

There were 885,000 new unemployment claims last week and twenty million still receiving benefits through one of the pandemic relief programs. Many extended benefit programs are scheduled to expire at the end of the month unless Congress passes another stimulus bill in the next few days, which is unlikely.

DECEMBER 18, 2020

2,794 COVID deaths in 24 hours
114,751 people in hospitals with COVID

The vaccine by Moderna was approved for emergency use by the FDA today, which will increase the number of vaccine doses for distribution in the US and around the world. The Pfizer and Moderna vaccines are similar with better than 90% effectiveness using the new mRNA technology.

The challenge now is distribution. Given the weather, and the holiday mail rush hampered by election damage, and the attempt by the wealthy to bribe their way to the head of the line, the rollout is just about as smooth as expected. And since the time needed for quality control was not included in the original timetable, we are behind delivery projections.

The vaccine represents a bright star in a dark night that seems a billion miles away for most of us. Even with priority for the elderly, our turn is still months away. The US may see half a million new cases each day before then and spend several more months in quarantine and isolation.

December 19, 2020

2,610 COVID deaths in 24 hours
113,929 people in hospitals with COVID

The UK is in emergency lockdown due to a new strain of the virus that is 70% more transmissible than the original. The new variant was discovered in September and accounted for nearly 60% of the infections in the UK by mid-December. Christmas commerce has been canceled and the European Union (EU) has closed their border with the UK.

Every country in the EU is now monitoring virus infections to find evidence of the mutation. The new variant has been detected in a handful of countries, but it is too soon to track how and where it originated. So far, this mutation does not appear to be more deadly—or immune to the new vaccines—but infection rates in the UK have doubled in a week.

In other news, Trump held a meeting with advisors in the White House yesterday, including several of the more controversial lawyers who suggested the following solutions to his election loss now that no court in the country has sided with him: He could confiscate election machines and show they have been altered; he could declare martial law and redo the election; he could use the military to force an outcome that allows him to stay.

There are first-person accounts of shouting matches in the Oval Office, but everyday Americans barely react to a possible coup at the highest level of our government. Future students (and their children and grandchildren) will research this time of compounding threats to the survival of the nation—a pandemic, an economic collapse, a racial injustice reckoning, an attempted presidential coup—and be inspired by our resilience. Hopefully.

The kids arrived at nine pm after sixteen hours on the road. They reported being shocked to see so few people with masks in Wyoming and Idaho and were as quick with their stops as humanly possible. My prediction of a lonely Christmas was entirely incorrect.

DECEMBER 21, 2020

1,841 COVID deaths in 24 hours

Thirty nations have closed their doors to travelers from the UK, including Austria, Belgium, Bulgaria, France, Germany, Ireland, Italy, and the Netherlands; other nations have some restrictions, including Canada, India, Iran, and Russia; a few are now closed to international travel, including Israel and South Africa. The governor of New York has requested a new travel ban into East Coast airports from Europe but also admits it could be too late to stop the new strain in the US.

There were more than a million travelers a day through US airports over the past three days, a record this year. Most will rejoin families without a quarantine and then return to their homes and jobs, also without a quarantine. And in South Dakota the anti-mask policy of the governor has led to the death of more nursing-home patients per capita than in any state in the US. They are tied with Sweden for the win in the "hang-out-the-elders-to-dry" category.

In Oregon, an armed mob of "Patriot Boys" stormed the capital while legislators were in closed session discussing mitigation efforts in the state. They were maskless, carried US and MAGA flags, and automatic weapons. They were met by Capitol police in riot gear, which was confusing since these boys also marched to "Back the Blue" during the race riots last summer. "No more blue support!" they shouted when the police pushed back. Approximately three hundred confused and angry protestors were dispersed in two hours, but not before a few roamed the halls of the Oregon State Capitol with assault weapons.

In the good news category, 614,000 people in the US have received COVID vaccines and Saturn and Jupiter are aligned—a conjunction—for the first time in eight hundred years.

DECEMBER 22, 2020

3,376 COVID deaths in 24 hours

Even at the end of the road in Wallowa County, a hundred Moderna vaccine doses were delivered which will be used to protect the hospital and clinic employees and other front-line workers. Tens of thousands of Christmas packages have not been delivered due to the backlog at the post office, but the vaccine got through, which inspires hope.

We are hugging and eating and drinking here at Angelkeep…all together for the first time since last Christmas. Everyone is in a festive mood, especially since Rachel and Kevin announced they are expecting a baby in July. Perhaps the very first reader for whom this journal is intended is on the way.

DECEMBER 23, 2020

3,401 COVID deaths in 24 hours

Travelers from the UK brought the more transmissible strain of the COVID virus during holiday travel to nearly a dozen countries including France, Spain, Japan, Italy, Germany, Lebanon, Sweden, Netherlands, Belgium and Australia so far. The US now requires proof of a negative COVID test before citizens of the UK can board a plane for the states. There is some concern that the surge in California may be related to the new variant.

It is expected that COVID reporting will be slowed by the holiday and not reflect accurate numbers for infection, hospitalization, or death for a week at least.

DECEMBER 24, 2020

2,835 COVID deaths in 24 hours
120,000 people in hospitals with COVID

There are 337,066 additional empty chairs at Christmas Eve dinner tonight in American homes; three hundred thousand more than the usual number of loved ones who die from disease and accidents in a normal year. Our hearts are with those who are grieving.

DECEMBER 26, 2020

As expected, President Trump is issuing dozens of pardons and commutations to anyone who is friendly to him including four military contractors who murdered Iraqis, a dozen white collar crooks including his daughter's father-in-law, Republican representatives and senators who are guilty of insider trading, friends who defrauded Medicare…and lots of tax cheats (after his own heart).

The stimulus bill is now stalled due to Trump's criticism of the checks to individuals…and the Republicans who negotiated on his behalf have been thrown under the bus. Trump tweeted that $600 is a disgrace and people should receive $2000 each.

No one really knows what happens next since Trump is golfing in Florida, but he may not sign the carefully-crafted compromise this year. What we do know is that fourteen million people have exhausted their unemployment benefits as of today and there is no hope in sight.

DECEMBER 28, 2020

Although twenty million doses of vaccine are available, the plan to distribute the vaccine is failing due to a lack of planning and funding at the federal level. Only eleven million doses have been received by the states and only two million have been administered, mostly to healthcare workers. Again, Trump deflects blame, saying it is up to the states to administer the vaccine, an excuse we have heard before.

"It is up to the states" was the excuse for the lack of federal planning for testing and for contact tracing and for providing PPE to frontline workers; "It is up to the states" was the excuse for a lack of national mask mandates and business closures that would have mitigated the spread. At every turn, the Trump administration has abdicated its responsibility for the safety of the people. At the current rate, it would take several years to reach the 80% vaccination rate required to stop the virus.

Luckily, President-elect Biden has said that fighting the virus will be the top priority for the first hundred days of his presidency. He will focus on getting a hundred million doses of the vaccine produced and administered and ask everyone in the nation to mask-up for a hundred days, which is a bridge too far for half of us. January 20 cannot come soon enough.

DECEMBER 30, 2020

	CASES	DEATHS	DEATHS/MILLION	DAILY NEW
WORLD:	83,055,202	1,811,358	232	728,653
US:	20,217,241	350,780	1,057	234,775

Both the deaths and hospitalizations reported today are record highs as expected. And these numbers do not reflect the post-holiday surge expected in two or three weeks since millions traveled during the holiday.

The UK variant was confirmed in Colorado when two National Guard soldiers infected all the residents and staff of a nursing home where they were sent to serve. It is not entirely clear if they caught the variant there or brought it with them.

They have no ICU beds available in California, so ambulances sit in bays waiting for someone to die before they can offload patients. There are few remaining oxygen tanks and the morgues are overflowing. The governor has issued a stay-at-home order for most of the state. There is concern that the variant is causing uncontrolled spread of the virus but crowding and poverty are primary factors with nearly half the dead among the those living in multi-generational housing.

DECEMBER 31, 2020

3,438 COVID deaths in 24 hours
125,379 people in hospitals with COVID

It is New Year's Eve and there will be no crowds to watch the big ball drop in Times Square, an event that has drawn massive crowds to mark the final moments of every year since 1904—except twice during the Second World War when it was also not safe to gather so closely together.

The vaccine rollout is a failure so far and heartbreaking to witness. Less than three million people have been vaccinated in the past two weeks although eleven million doses have been shipped. There is confusion among the nation's healthcare workers about who to vaccinate, and how to store and distribute the vaccine.

There was sabotage of a vaccine supply by an anti-vaxxer, and so much misinformation online that entire healthcare teams and nursing home staffs have refused to take the vaccine. Some doses will expire before an efficient delivery system is established in each state. Once again, without leadership we are failing.

Trump is still trying to overturn the election. His latest and most desperate act is to force Republican representatives and at least one senator to vote against certifying election results on January 6—a pro forma constitutional exercise. House leaders required a debate about voter fraud even though no court or state has found any evidence of fraud...not a shred of evidence. The sycophants participating in this coup attempt are putting their political future ahead of the nation and practicing sedition to gain power. Will there be consequences?

Meanwhile, Wall Street finished the year at a record high after a record loss in March, minting fifty-six new billionaires while tens of millions were left unemployed and hungry and waiting in long lines at the food bank to survive.

One of the worst years in American history comes to an end at midnight. Good riddance to 2020 and (hopefully) to the worst president in American history.

JANUARY 2, 2021

There are now eleven Republican senators who have announced they plan to vote against certifying the election even though the President-elect Biden won by a margin of nearly eight million votes and seventy-four electors. And there are 146 Republican representatives who will also vote against certifying the electors despite having lost nearly sixty legal challenges. And there are millions of Americans who are convinced there was fraud due to constant messaging from the outgoing president that he won the election. He is manufacturing an alternative reality for economic profit and political power.

Imagine any athlete of any age in any sport trying to overturn the results of a game everyone watched by jumping up and down and screaming, "But I won!" These Republicans have sided with their dear leader—with his tantrums and treason—over the health and welfare of the nation by denying the legitimacy of a fair election, the same election responsible for hundreds of Republican wins.

Finer minds assure us that the coup will fail but this "win at any cost" philosophy of partisan politics is suppressing our democracy just as the "profit at any cost" ideology of vulture capitalism is strangling our economy.

Neither vaccination nor a soaring stock market will solve the problem of selfishness that is plaguing our country. Americans really need to grow up.

JANUARY 3, 2021

One year ago, the WHO reported that there was an unusual cluster of pneumonia in Wuhan, China—with forty-four cases and no deaths—via a tweet. Two weeks later a US citizen returned from the province and became the first COVID case recorded in the US, although there is some indication that the virus was circulating in California a month earlier.

One year later, the US has not controlled the pandemic, with hundreds of thousands of new cases a day, tens of thousands of deaths each week, and a hospital system near the brink of collapse. And still, 2.5 million people flew home from holiday gatherings this weekend.

The new Congress was seated today, with 140 Republican members still planning to contest the outcome of the election on January 6, the same election in which they acquired their seat. One still wonders how these newly elected leaders can swear an oath and cry fraud at the same time.

Trump still thinks he can change the outcome as reflected in a recorded phone call to the Secretary of State in Georgia. Trump is heard arguing against known facts, desperately pleading to "find" 11,000 votes, and indirectly threatening the secretary to change the results to reflect his "win," a violation of the federal extortion laws. Many have called for an investigation into his coup attempt but a dozen senators—now called the dirty dozen—still plan to vote against confirming the legal winner of the electoral college when they meet on Wednesday.

Trump has issued a call to the Proud Boys and all supporting right-wing militias that it's time to stand forward…to gather in Washington DC on January 6 to protest the stolen election. One congressman even suggested it was time for violence; the National Guard has apparently been activated.

The intimidation of election officials in Georgia is partly due to the Senate runoff election on Tuesday—the outcome of this election for Georgia's two open seats will determine the Senate majority. There has never been a more consequential runoff election in a state so closely divided: once reliably red, the capital city of Atlanta is now turning blue.

Hundreds of millions have been spent on these two runoff races. Accusations of fraud are being levied by Trump and his supporters because Black Americans are voting in unprecedented numbers; voter suppression tactics are no longer working in Georgia.

This is a defining week for our country. Will we tolerate Trump promoting a coup in plain sight? Will Congress—and the Republican party—tear itself apart over the issue? Will there be violence on the streets of DC? Will the Senate change hands and give Democrats the power to lead? Stay tuned.

JANUARY 4, 2021

England announced a third national lockdown to manage soaring new infections caused by a highly-transmissible variant. All nonessential workers are required to stay in their homes except to purchase groceries and medicine or to exercise outdoors. Daycares and churches are open, but restaurants and bars and all schools are closed until mid-February. Scotland has also returned to lockdown after a Christmas easing of restrictions, with Ireland soon to follow due to a dramatic surge in cases.

The new variant has now been reported in four US states—Colorado, California, Florida and New York—which is of grave concern to public health officials because we could soon experience a variant surge upon a holiday surge upon a winter surge—a triple threat.

In Los Angeles County, a human disaster is unfolding, and the county is pleading for help. They recently asked the Army Corp of Engineers to install additional oxygen capacity in the hospitals because outdated lines were freezing up with overuse. The county supervisor sent a letter to the governor requesting that the hospital ship USNS *Mercy* return to the Port of Los Angeles and provide emergency support for their overwhelmed hospital system.

And due to a continuing lack of beds at every ICU in LA, county leaders have told emergency workers to transport only those with a chance of survival. Heart attack and gunshot victims and anyone else too sick to survive can only be treated on-site.

With a 20% positivity rate and record-high hospitalizations, the LA pandemic will get worse before it gets better. This surge was created by Thanksgiving gatherings; the surge from Christmas travel and New Year's Eve celebrations and the new variant will arrive at the end of the month.

And still—in the middle of an escalating health disaster—virus deniers in LA are terrorizing their neighbors. With lethal irony, a gang without masks descended on Westfield Century City Mall yesterday and harassed the shoppers who were wearing masks. These anti-maskers were spitting and screaming about personal freedom, putting everyone within range of their tantrum at risk.

JANUARY 5, 2020

Finally, the press and politicians are calling Trump's efforts to overturn the election what it is: a coup attempt supported by congressional sycophants who have political ambitions. The streets of DC have filled with supporters encouraged by the president to protest the "stolen election."

After a long day of voting in Georgia, a Democratic preacher, Raphael Warnock, who currently leads the historic Martin Luther King congregation, won a Senate seat from an incumbent Republican whose spouse—Chair of the New York Stock Exchange—contributed twenty-one million dollars to her failed campaign.

And even more surprising is that a 33-year-old documentary filmmaker, Jon Ossoff, is on his way to winning the second Georgia Senate seat from a Republican incumbent and flip the Senate to Democratic control. Conservative Republicans blame Trump's coup attempt for the loss of these two seats and the Senate.

Tomorrow, during the ceremonial certification of the presidential election, Republicans will need to decide if they are with the president's coup attempt or against it; they will need to decide if they will uphold the Constitution or ignore it. With two Democratic wins in Georgia, lying to Congress for the sake of power looks like a fool's errand.

President Trump's legacy is confirmed: In his four disastrous years he lost the presidency, his party's control of the House of Representatives and the US Senate, tens of millions of jobs, and 348,330 American lives due to his incompetence during the pandemic.

JANUARY 6, 2021

This day will forever be remembered as the Day of Insurrection in the United States. Eight thousand Trump supporters—including members of White supremacy militias—listened to his call to stop the vote in Congress, marched down Pennsylvania Avenue after his incendiary speech, and stormed into the Capitol Building; they destroyed offices, furniture and precious artwork, and threatened House and Senate members who were certifying the election. "Stop the Steal!" was chanted. They carried zip ties, metal pipes, helmets, bats and stun guns in a premeditated attack planned on social media.

The US Capitol Building is the beacon of democracy for the world, for the nation, and for the American citizens who consider it "the people's house," and it was somehow easily overrun by a mob who believe the election was stolen. Trump retreated to the White House cafeteria and reportedly enjoyed watching the crisis unfold on TV. For three long hours he refused to call for the immediate cessation of violence, and then congratulated the mob and expressed his "love" for them when he addressed the nation that afternoon.

Members of Congress were either moved to a secret location—including the vice president—or barricaded in place under desks and benches while clutching or wearing gas masks. Guns were drawn, tear gas was used, and four people died during the insurrection, something that has not happened inside the Capitol since 1812. The nation—and the world—watched as the destruction unfolded in real time. After control was regained, Congress resumed deliberations—with some STILL declaring fraud—and certified the election.

Even though there are only fourteen days left in this presidency, there are calls for a second impeachment. Some suggest invoking the 25th Amendment to remove Trump from office for inciting a riot against the US Capitol and Congress. Members of his administration are resigning in protest, leaders of the party are issuing scathing public criticism, and the FBI is conducting a nationwide search for those who broke windows and doors to gain access, breached the walls with ropes, swarmed the rotunda, debased our national treasures, roamed the halls looking for targets, raised Confederate flags in victory and used flagpoles as weapons.

The major social media sites have all suspended Trump's accounts to silence his continued claims that the election was stolen and to limit his ability to mobilize supporters. Afterward, on camera, his supporters pledged to return with guns.

Four years ago, President Trump gave an inaugural speech that included the threat of "American Carnage" and today we saw what he meant. He also stoked carnage during a pandemic—causing death and destruction—and the world is watching.

I was wrong to blithely assume there would be a peaceful transition of power—the hallmark of US democracy—and now we wonder how to survive the final fourteen days. The Republican party is at war with itself, and the nation is suffering the consequences. This presidency is ending with violence that has shocked the nation—violence Trump encouraged, violence that now defines his legacy.

JANUARY 7, 2021

4,033 COVID deaths in 24 hours, a record

"Resign or be impeached a second time." This refrain from the pages of the nation's most conservative newspapers, business organizations, former cabinet members, and evangelical leaders who invested him with nearly divine power for political purposes, signals a universal condemnation of the insurrection against the US Capitol led by Trump and his MAGA followers.

Speaker McCarthy called the Chairman of the Joint Chiefs to ask what tools are available to stop a mentally unstable and obviously unfit president with the nuclear codes from doing any more damage during the next thirteen days. Articles of impeachment will be ready for a vote next week, the only time in the nation's history a president has been impeached twice.

Meanwhile, daily deaths from COVID surpass four thousand for the first time, hospitalizations are still at record highs, and the surge continues due to the rapid spread of the variant. Hospital triage plans have been implemented in Los Angeles, with "triage officers" evaluating who can be saved and then ending emergency care for those who can't. The death rate is doubling.

Although vaccine rollout is slow, Keith was able to receive his first Moderna dose today due to his role as Public Health Officer in Union County. Because of the rapidly spreading surge of infection, President-elect Biden has decided that most of the available vaccines should be distributed now instead of being held back for second doses. He still promises to distribute a hundred million doses in his first hundred days.

JANUARY 8, 2021

How is it possible that an angry mob was able to penetrate the US Capitol without encountering strong barriers and a police presence? The threat of violence on January 6 was broadcast widely on social media and encouraged by the president. Was there inside help?

A photograph of a Capitol police officer posing for a selfie with insurgents has raised questions, but the small Capitol police force tried to protect and serve. One member of the force died after being bludgeoned with a fire extinguisher. Three Capitol police leaders who are tasked with protecting the US Capitol Building and the Congress and the Senate have resigned, and an investigation is pending.

The Capitol police response to White supremacy insurgents this week, and the federal troop response to Black Lives Matter protesters last June at Lafayette Square—when police in riot gear tear-gassed and pepper-sprayed peaceful Black Lives Matter protestors to clear the square—provides evidence of a serious double standard for policing based on race. As one commenter put it: "When Black people are protesting it is called violence; when White people are violent it is called protesting."

Articles of Impeachment will be introduced in the House on Monday and there are enough votes for impeachment. The Senate leader, Mitch McConnell, has said they will not take up the question until after the inauguration of the president-elect, but with the new Democratic majority, it is possible the Senate will at least vote to restrict the current president from holding any office in the US ever again.

Twitter permanently banned Trump due to continued tweets about election fraud and his willingness to incite violence. Unfortunately, there are indications on multiple social media platforms that the president's anarchists are planning further violence prior to January 20. The Proud Boys are again "standing by" and will likely step out again as White nationalist traitors to the nation.

In other news, after seven months of job gains there were 140,000 jobs lost in December and nearly 800,000 new unemployment claims filed last week.

JANUARY 10, 2021

As expected, people are becoming agitated about when the vaccine will be available to the public. Here in Oregon, medical and behavioral health workers and nursing-home residents can receive a shot but the roll-out is so slow they have expanded distribution criteria to speed up the process. The CDC today said anyone over sixty-five should receive a shot. Every day, there are record-high infections, hospitalizations, and deaths; the Christmas surge is here.

The extent of the violence on January 6 is becoming increasingly clear. There are videos of insurrectionists grabbing police officers and beating them with flagpoles or pushing them through doorways as they tried to rush the Senate chambers. Unfortunately, there is also video evidence showing Capitol police officers offering encouragement to the rioters—two officers were suspended and another dozen are under investigation.

The FBI issued an internal memo on January 5 warning of "war" at the Capitol but did not share the brief with Capitol police. Now the FBI has issued a public warning that violence is expected again in Washington DC and in all fifty state capitals before or during the inauguration; the White supremacy militias who are supported by the president have threatened to continue their "civil war."

Accountability for the "stolen election" lie is rising since social media companies are cracking down on widespread misinformation; corporations are holding back contributions to those who supported the lie; banks are ending relationships with Trump and his Foundation; the PGA pulled its major events from his golf clubs. But still, many Republican politicians repeat the lie because their supporters have already been brainwashed.

There must be a sea-change regarding truth in the nation, a reckoning of the danger we face when leaders use misinformation as a political tool and people believe them.

JANUARY 12, 2021

Since COVID infections are followed by hospitalizations which are followed by deaths, there have been record number of deaths three weeks after the Christmas holiday. At the current rate, we will see nearly 100,000 deaths from COVID during the month of January 2021, currently the leading cause of death in the US.

Amid sedition and insurrection and impeachment, it is almost impossible to focus clearly on the human tragedy unfolding in the nation's hospitals, but one commentator clearly summed up the pain:

"One of the more heartbreaking conversations that our healthcare workers share is about these last words when children apologize to their parents and grandparents for bringing COVID into their homes, for getting them sick," Los Angeles County Supervisor Hilda Solis said.

These final conversations are happening on the phone or tablet screens that the nurses hold near the dying so these last words can be heard amid the beeps and alarms and whirring of machines.

There is an unprecedented national manhunt for those who participated in the Capitol insurrection. The FBI is sifting through a massive amount of digital evidence that was posted on social media during the riot and matching faces with names. Pictures are being released with requests for help identifying people and a hotline for tips has received over 120,000 responses.

In addition, police, fire, and military organizations are combing the same evidence to identify participants from their own ranks, and there are many. The history of the police force is linked to White nationalism since it was originally used to control slaves in the south and immigrants in the north. It is no surprise that the White supremacy movement attracts those with police and military backgrounds.

The Joint Chiefs in charge of the military felt compelled to issue a strong statement to condemn "sedition and insurrection" and remind all troops that they have sworn an oath to defend the Constitution.

"*We witnessed actions inside the Capitol building that were inconsistent with the rule of law. The rights of freedom of speech and assembly do not give anyone the right to resort to violence, sedition and insurrection,*" said the statement, released Tuesday and signed by America's most senior general, Mark Milley, and the entire Joint Chiefs of Staff, which is comprised of the heads of each military branch.

Tomorrow, the US House of Representatives will vote on the single article of impeachment against the president, which reads:

"*President Trump gravely endangered the security of the United States and its institutions of Government. He threatened the integrity of the democratic system, interfered with the peaceful transition of power, and imperiled a coequal branch of Government. He thereby betrayed his trust as President, to the manifest injury of the people of the United States.*"

Today each representative was able to speak for thirty seconds "for" or "against" impeachment; simultaneously, someone in the nation died of COVID every twenty seconds due to an uncontrolled virus that will kill half a million Americans before we find the will to stop it.

The virus of White nationalism and the COVID virus are both deadly threats to the nation. Both must be identified and eliminated.

JANUARY 14, 2021

Rep. Liz Cheney, third highest Republican in the House of Representatives, voted for impeachment of the president, writing: "*The President of the United States summoned this mob, assembled this mob, and lit the flame of this attack. There has never been a greater betrayal by a president of the United States of his office and his oath to the Constitution.*"

Final vote: 232 in favor, including ten Republicans for and 197 against. Trump has been impeached for a second time in his one-term presidency. The Senate will hold the trial of the president after the inauguration on January 20.

President-elect Biden addressed the nation to outline the $1.9 trillion "American Rescue Plan" that he will begin implementing next week. He started by reviewing the economic facts of the American economy due to the pandemic: Fourteen million households are behind on rent; one in seven households do not have enough to eat, including thirty million adults and twelve million children; eighteen million are still receiving unemployment benefits; 400,000 small businesses have closed their doors.

He also reminded us that fifty percent of the top corporations have added trillions in profit during the pandemic and ninety of the nation's largest corporations paid no income tax in 2019. He pledges to make sure everyone pays their fair share of taxes going forward. He will raise the minimum wage to $15 saying "no one working 40 hours per week should be living below the poverty line."

Last week there were 1.4 million new unemployment claims, including 965,000 regular claims and over 400,000 for pandemic unemployment provided by the federal government to the self-employed.

The state of Oregon opened vaccinations to all those over sixty-five years of age following the recommendation of the CDC, and I am scheduled for my first dose on January 19, the day before the inauguration.

JANUARY 15, 2021

	Cases	Deaths	Daily new	Daily deaths
World:	93,851,000	2,009,000	740,083	14,645
US:	23,600,000	399,600	243,996	3,679

True to form, the Trump administration lied to the American people when it announced that the second doses held in reserve would all be released and everyone over sixty-five would be vaccinated. There were no second doses held in reserve and we will not get the vaccine next week…or likely the week after. The angry reaction from governors was swift, and the disappointment among those sixty-five and older is profound, including my own, although I have little to complain about compared to most.

For ten months the newly-retired have been isolated at home, unable to see friends or family, to shop and travel or attend the normal celebrations of a well-lived life. Many have had as much loneliness as they can handle and see their remaining time slipping away.

Although the 65+ age group has had only 17% of the infections, they have suffered 90% of the deaths. My age group cannot afford to take any chances and are captive at home and isolated from friends until we receive the vaccine. Last year at this time we were packing suitcases for a trip to Hawaii with our newly widowed best friend, and this year we are watching unrelenting virus death and race riots and insurrection every night on cable news and dreaming of freedom.

President-elect Biden presented his new vaccination plan, and it appears robust: FEMA and the National Guard will assume the vaccination logistics role, setting up vaccination centers and distributing supplies. Building the infrastructure is a critical next step but the real problem is the shortage of vaccine. Where is all the vaccine? Everyone is pondering the same thing since Trump bragged about getting millions of doses to Americans in record time.

And now, public health officials are warning that a highly transmissible variant already detected in fifty countries could become dominant in the US by March, a possibility with deadly consequences. January may not be the worst month of the pandemic if infection rates rapidly rise in the next two months. We are now neck-and-neck in a race with a mutating virus—an already long marathon that can only be won with new leadership and unlimited resources.

JANUARY 17, 2021

There are 25,000 National Guard troops with pistols and rifles stationed around the Capitol in advance of the inauguration on Wednesday. There are miles of fencing topped with barbed-wire, tanks and armored cars, barricades and checkpoints. It looks like a war zone. The city is shut-down, Airbnb and travel hotels have cancelled all bookings for the week, the airlines are refusing to check luggage with weapons; every insurrectionist identified so far has been added to the no-fly list.

Two months of lies amplified on social media has convinced 74% of the Republican party that the election was rigged. To curry favor, elected officials continued to amplify Trump's lies and a great mass hysteria has been firmly seated in the Republican mind. Even after sixty failed lawsuits and a deadly insurrection that threatened the US Congress, the Big Lie persists.

But the problem is bigger than the lie. It appears that the insurrection was planned in the White House and executed by White supremacists who have recruited members from the military and the police force. Background checks are underway for the 25,000 troops that are currently surrounding the White House and Capitol buildings.

JANUARY 18, 2021

There are now four COVID variants that scientists are watching: B.1.1.7 from the UK that is now present in fifty countries and twenty US states; B.1.351 from South Africa that is now the dominant strain in several African countries; P.1 and P.2 in Brazil that are reinfecting areas that have already experienced a surge; and L452R in California that is present in 25% of the state's infections. It is surmised that the UK variant and the California variant have been circulating in the US for months, but genomic testing for variants has been slow.

Mutations occur with great frequency, an evolutionary tool for the "natural selection" of strengths needed for living organisms to adapt to a changing environment. With increasing antibodies from infection and vaccines, the virus has a less friendly environment to reproduce; mutations that boost transmission rates will produce variants that thrive.

Epidemiologists believe that these variants are not a threat to the effectiveness of the vaccines since the human immune system adapts well to viral mutations. However, as the pool of hosts continues to diminish over the next few years and the virus adapts, the vaccines will need to be updated. We can expect that we will need annual COVID shots just as we need annual flu shots to keep up with variants.

We are nearing 400,000 deaths from COVID and we will likely reach half a million deaths before March, before vaccines begin to slow the current surge of infection.

The one-year anniversary of the first COVID case confirmed in the US happens to coincide with the inauguration of our new president—January 20th—a president who recognizes the lethality of the virus and will provide competent leadership...finally.

JANUARY 20, 2021

4,409 COVID deaths in 24 hours, another record

It is hard to express how excited I am about today's inaugural events. I rose from a restless night at 5:30 am to watch the departure of the outgoing president and his family on Air Force One as they left the White House and headed to their golf club in Florida.

Ex-President Trump did not concede the election or call to congratulate the new president or invite President Biden and his wife to tour the White House or ride with him to the inauguration as is customary. And he is not attending the inauguration today, a tradition that has been in place for 150 years, a tradition that represents the peaceful transition of power in this nation. In keeping with his entire presidency, this historic snub will be remembered for another 150 years—ex-president Trump has displayed a complete lack of dignity and grace.

At the same time, a great weight was lifted as that plane carrying the worst president in US history taxied and circled and flew away south.

The new president was sworn in at noon, flanked by both Republicans and Democrats, which was reassuring since they stood together on the same steps where a deadly mob of Trump insurrectionists had attempted to overthrow the government two weeks earlier. It was reassuring to see every leader from the three branches of government gather to transfer power from one administration to another...every leader except the one who incited a riot to try and force himself upon the country for another four years.

The first woman vice president in history, a Black woman of Asian descent, was escorted to the podium by the Black Capitol police officer whose actions saved the Senate from being overrun during the riot.

President Joe Biden, who has served in the US Senate and as vice president during fifty years of public service, pledged himself to unity and promised to do everything in his power to control this deadly pandemic.

It is a new day in a new era. We watch with tears of joy as our nation rises—with one giant step—from the ashes. In the words of our new president, "Democracy has prevailed!"

Part Four: Vaccines and Variants

January 21-February 26, 2021

JANUARY 21, 2021

President Biden held a press conference from the Oval Office to discuss his administration's COVID strategy which was published on the whitehouse.gov website and is 198 pages in length.

He was candid, saying "Things will get worse before they get better." He likened the COVID fight to a war and reminded us that we have lost as many people in ten months as we did in four years during WWII. "Of course this is a war," he said, calling the pandemic a national emergency and warning of another 100,000 dead next month.

President Biden announced that the US has rejoined the World Health Organization and will provide funding and expertise, with Dr. Anthony Fauci representing the US. He has again promised to vaccinate a hundred million Americans in the first one hundred days of his administration.

To accomplish the vaccination task, he will authorize FEMA to set up one hundred vaccination centers, authorize the CDC to develop and oversee a pharmacy vaccination plan, expand the pool of professionals needed to administer vaccines by recruiting retired healthcare workers, reimburse states for National Guard expenses, and require insurance companies to provide free COVID testing.

As promised, President Biden signed the following ten Executive Orders today (as summarized in *USA Today*, 1/21/21):

- Direct federal agencies to exercise all appropriate authorities, including invoking the Defense Production Act, to accelerate manufacturing and delivery to meet shortfalls in equipment and supplies to respond to the COVID-19 pandemic.
- Establish the COVID-19 Pandemic Testing Board to bring the "full force of the federal government's expertise" to expanding testing supply and increasing access to testing. The order directs federal agencies to facilitate testing free for those who lack health insurance and to clarify insurers' obligation to cover testing.
- Direct new studies—including large-scale randomized trials—to identify treatments for COVID-19 with a focus on addressing the needs of diverse populations. The order will direct federal agencies to expand their data infrastructure to increase the collection and sharing of data to support an equitable COVID-19 response and recovery.
- Direct "a national strategy for safely reopening schools," including requiring the Education and Health and Human Services departments to provide guidance on the safe reopening and operating of schools, childcare providers and higher education institutions.
- Require masks be worn in airports and certain modes of transportation such as planes, trains, maritime vessels and intercity buses.
- Establish a COVID-19 Health Equity Task Force to provide recommendations to the president for allocating resources and funding in communities with inequities in COVID-19 outcomes by race, ethnicity, disability and other considerations.

- Restore full federal reimbursement to states and tribes—up from 75%—for National Guard personnel and emergency supplies, as well as equipment and manpower for vaccination centers.
- Direct the Occupational Safety and Health Administration to issue updated guidance on COVID-19 worker protections.
- Improve access to COVID-19 care and treatment. That includes outlining steps to bolster clinical care capacity, assist long-term care facilities and facilities for people with disabilities, increase health care workforce capacity and support access to COVID-19 therapies for the uninsured.
- Direct the restoration of America's leadership globally to support the "international pandemic response effort." The directive supports the international health and humanitarian response to the COVID-19 pandemic.

In a subsequent press conference, Dr. Fauci responded to a question regarding his new boss by saying, "The idea that I can get up here and state what I know—to use expertise and science—is liberating." The new press secretary promised daily briefings and in a first for the nation, President Biden elevated his science advisor—who is director of the Office of Science and Technology Policy—to a cabinet level position. He has promised to lead using the best science available.

JANUARY 22, 2020

Instead of balls and parades and a capital city swarming with citizens, the Biden inauguration was subject to the social distancing and security checkpoints required by a raging pandemic and civil unrest.

And still, it was one of the more uplifting days I can remember: There were ceremonies designed to help us grieve the loss of 400,000 loved ones; happy speeches and a heartfelt poem that challenged us to be better—to do better; an "American Celebration" that showcased talented musicians, including A-list stars performing on the steps of the Lincoln Memorial framed by four hundred memorial lanterns that shimmered along the Reflecting Pool all the way to the Washington Monument.

It felt like America turned 180 degrees in 24 hours, banished a mean alter-ego, and embraced what the dream of unity might look like going forward. I will never forget President Biden and the First Lady standing on the White House balcony with fireworks bursting in every direction, surrounding them. The entire day was breathtakingly beautiful.

JANUARY 23, 2021

We are seeing the consequences of the previous administration's lack of a vaccine distribution plan: complete chaos. The current administration incorrectly assumed there was a plan that had not been forwarded to the incoming administration for political reasons, but no federal plan existed except the CDC recommendations for priorities.

All fifty states are having problems, each with different rules, priorities, protocols and resources needed to get the vaccine into the arms of desperate Americans. Most vaccination centers do not know how much vaccine they will have day to day, so appointments are made and cancelled by the thousands which leaves people frantic to reschedule and frustrated trying to navigate crowded websites and phone lines—a veritable "Hunger Games" for vaccine access.

And, of course, there are stories of people cheating and stealing and flying to Florida from Venezuela to get a shot; there are wealthy people offering donations and cash payments to concierge medical practices. The governors of New York and California have threatened penalties for "line-skipping."

Although the CDC has prioritized people over the age of 65, here in Oregon the governor has prioritized teachers, childcare providers, and essential workers ahead of the elderly, a policy many support. It will be another month before those 65+ will have access to the vaccine in Oregon but the children can safely return to school.

Across the US, forty-four million doses of the vaccine have been delivered but only eighteen million have been administered leading many to wonder where all the doses are and why they have not been used when so many people are waiting to be vaccinated. Hopefully, the new focus on vaccine manufacturing and distribution—and federal financial support for the states—will greatly increase the number of vaccinations completed, meeting the goal of one hundred million in the first one hundred days.

JANUARY 25, 2021

As of tomorrow, all travelers to the US will need proof of a negative COVID test seventy-two hours before boarding the plane, no exceptions.

"As variants of the SARS-CoV-2 virus continue to emerge in countries around the world, there is growing evidence of increased transmissibility of some of these variants, as well as unknown health and vaccine implications," a CDC spokesman said in a statement. "Testing before and after travel is a critical layer to slow the introduction and spread of COVID-19 and emerging variants."

Although it looks as if the holiday surge is abating, fear of the variants is ramping up. There are known cases of all four variants in the US and efforts to test the vaccines against variants are underway, especially the South African strain which appears to lower antibody protection. Dr. Fauci suggests that a booster shot may be needed. In the meantime, the CDC recommends people wear double masks for added protection. Due to her pregnancy, we encouraged Rachel to wear the N95 mask in the medical kit we sent last March if she spends any time with people other than family indoors.

The variants are causing havoc in the rest of the world as well. The UK remains in lockdown due to recent news that the variant could be more deadly than the original virus. The Netherlands and Israel are experiencing riots in response to new restrictions after discovering the UK variant, and Denmark is seeing a 70% rise each week in variant cases due to thorough genomic testing—the best in the world—which proves the variants are spreading rapidly.

The good news is that another vaccine from Johnson & Johnson may be approved for emergency use in the next two weeks. This new vaccine requires a single dose and easier storage, which makes for faster distribution. In addition, some trials were held in Brazil and South Africa, which might provide answers about effectiveness against the current variants. They will release findings in a few days and all fingers are crossed that we can add another vaccine to the world's pandemic arsenal. We are in a race with a wickedly agile predator.

JANUARY 27, 2021

There has been a 35% decline in new COVID infections in the past three weeks and fewer hospitalizations, which may point to a small step towards herd immunity after a year with rising infections.

It is estimated that there are three additional asymptomatic or mild cases for every one case reported, which means nearly a hundred million Americans have had some exposure and may have developed antibodies. In addition, nearly twenty-five million have received at least one vaccine, so a third of us—125 million—may have some protection from infection.

Unfortunately, these are also the same circumstances that give rise to new variants. With two-hundred million people in the US still without any protection, the virus can easily mutate into a new version of itself. Without adequate genome sequencing of the virus, it is impossible to tell how widespread the variants are or how many there are...or how long the current vaccines will be effective against them. We are nowhere near the end of this global pandemic.

JANUARY 28, 2021

Dr. Fauci warned that the spread of variants in the US, especially the South African variant known as B.1351, should be a wake-up call to vaccinate as many people as possible as quickly as possible. Many public health officials are now calling for more first-dose vaccinations instead of reserving second doses which they believe can be just as effective in the short term.

Although the Moderna and Pfizer vaccines are effective against most identified variants, they do not work as well against the B.1351 variant, and this has given rise to concern across the globe. New travel bans are in effect in Canada and the EU, requiring tests and quarantines before travelers are allowed into the countries, but B.1351 has been found in two dozen countries and a handful of states, so it cannot be stopped.

The Johnson & Johnson one-dose vaccine is only 57% effective against the B.1351 variant with an overall 66% effectiveness against the original virus, but it does help limit severe illness from COVID. The news has sent their stock value down and the market has dropped six hundred points today.

The International Labor Organization reported that 225 million jobs have been lost worldwide due to the pandemic, which is four times more jobs lost than during the great recession of 2009. They also reported that the top ten billionaires—who own social media and online shopping sites—gained enough in profit during the pandemic to vaccinate every person in the world.

In the US, more than a million new claims for unemployment were filed last week, which follows a trend upward since November 2020. The new administration is working on a stimulus package that may be the biggest in the nation's history. With Democrats in the majority in all three branches, the stimulus is likely to pass along party lines with a simple majority vote. Now that Republican leaders are in the minority, they are suddenly concerned about deficits, but the economic situation for more than half the nation is dire, and Democrats are moving full-steam ahead.

JANUARY 30, 2021

	Cases	Deaths	Daily new	Daily deaths
World:	102,584,000	2,220,000	514,496	13,524
US:	26,100,000	446,300	146,657	2,972

Twenty-two years ago, a British physician named Andrew Wakefield published a study, funded by a vaccine lawyer, that linked autism to MMR vaccines. The study was false—proven to be an outright fraud—but the myth lives on in the minds of those who are easily misled by manufactured outrage. They became the anti-vaxxers and are responsible for the online lies and misinformation that have put the world's children at risk from preventable disease.

The conspiracy-minded are having a field day with COVID vaccines and the lies are becoming more outrageous: They claim that it changes DNA and that the government (or Bill Gates) put microchips in the vaccine to track people. They have teamed up with the COVID deniers and the anti-maskers and the Stop the Stealers and the far-righters who do nothing but bully everyone unlike themselves.

A loose coalition of fifty hardliners shut down the vaccination center in Dodger Stadium for a few hours today, marching with signs that stated the pandemic is a hoax and the vaccines are dangerous. None were arrested but six thousand other people were forced to endure a much longer wait to receive a life-saving vaccine.

Some say that social media sites like Facebook and Twitter are responsible for letting lethal misinformation flourish on their sites, that they allow people to yell "FIRE!" in a crowded theater for profit. Is this free speech? Should someone who profits from misinformation be responsible for the results of that speech? What is the consequence for willfully turning people against life-saving science?

The only way to stop the virus is through herd immunity and the only way to reach herd immunity is through vaccines. The virus is mutating, and vaccinations will soon be less effective. We are in a race with the virus, but those who fear science are trying to trip us up…a classic battle with the evil of ignorance that good eventually wins.

FEBRUARY 1, 2021

On the other side of the good and evil question are those who justify skipping the line for a vaccine because they are willing to tell lies—instead of resisting good, they knowingly practice evil.

For example, there was a wealthy couple in Canada who flew to a remote village and posed as motel workers to receive shots intended for village elders; there was an online fitness instructor in New York who claimed she was a "teacher" and skipped the line even as thousands of real teachers had appointments canceled due to a lack of supply; there are tech savvy people traveling hours to poor neighborhoods where the online registration system was too complicated for the elderly and minorities to navigate without help.

And there are unending reports of outrageous profit being made while the world suffers and millions die, reports that question the success of human civilization. Profound moral and ethical questions always arise during times of sudden change, and the answers—by each person and family and business and country—defines success better than any balance sheet ever will.

It appears we have reached the apex of capitalism, where profit becomes more important than basic human need, an economic system that promotes personal wealth at the expense of progress for the whole. This object lesson in the consequences of selfishness may be the only medicine able to fight the virus of material greed and propel us forward—to evolve a world where all can survive….and thrive. How much suffering and death will we tolerate while personal profits soar?

FEBRUARY 3, 2021

Currently, vaccination appointments for the first dose are being cancelled or paused to ensure that second boosters are administered, which is incorrect according to some health experts who advocate prioritizing the first dose as a defense against rapidly spreading variants.

In Oregon, the governor has underestimated how many educators need vaccines and continues to push those 65 and older to the back of the line, although most states are vaccinating elders first. The wealthy and well-connected continue to line skip and it may be late spring before most of us can get out of the house; you can surely hear my frustration.

The Super Bowl will be held this weekend after a full season was played during the pandemic—minus fans in the stands. The economic consequences of missing a season forced the NFL to develop a robust COVID protocol for players, including continuous testing, contact tracing, and social distancing. They were so careful they could tell from genome sequencing the exact person who infected a particular player. Then they isolated a week or ten days and were back on the field; no serious illness has been reported. We should all play football.

FEBRUARY 9, 2021

35,000,000 COVID vaccines administered in the US

There were nine new cases in Wallowa County today, and twenty-seven new cases in the past nine days, bringing our total to 118 with 25% of the cases confirmed recently. Due to privacy issues and the fact that we have no public health agency here, information about how and where the rapid rise is occurring is left to rumor, but it seems a man with a temperature of 102 went to a school board meeting and infected his neighbors. He complained of feeling sick to the dismay of those in the room, and the school board meeting became a superspreader event.

The national numbers are more encouraging, with a 25% decline in cases and hospitalizations and deaths in the past week. The holiday surge is over, and the variant surge is yet to arrive, so we are in the eye of the storm. Public health officials still predict that the variant strain from the UK will be dominant in the US in another month.

The race to vaccinate ahead of the new strain is ongoing, but the pace of vaccinations is still slow due to inadequate supply and distribution protocols; the disparity in the rules from state to state has also caused frustration. In 26 states, teachers are prioritized over the elderly, and teachers' unions are suing in the 24 states that have prioritized the elderly. Most schools in populated areas still have no in-person classes.

The second impeachment trial of the ex-president for the January 6 insurrection began today with a dramatic opening video by the prosecution that reminded the nation of Trump's attempted coup. It is an historic event for the nation, with Republican senators refusing to acknowledge that the man who bullies them into compliance is also responsible for an attack on Congress. The trial is expected to continue for at least a week.

The current scene in the Senate Chambers—with everyone masked and socially distant—is surreal. Senators watch as rioters rifle through desks and surround the rostrum while shouting death threats and obscenities in their hallowed hall. They watch themselves cower behind chairs and under desks while the ex-president's supporters attack the police with flag poles and fire extinguishers. Currently the death toll stands at seven, including two officers who committed suicide, and 140 police wounded. More than two hundred insurgents have been arrested so far.

It is not likely they will reach a two-thirds majority for conviction, but the trial itself stands as a stark reminder of the consequences of allowing an unfit man to occupy the presidency. Hopefully, the grandchildren who might someday read this journal will study January 6, 2021, in their history books. We must never forget the danger and death that resulted from the worst presidency in American history.

FEBRUARY 11, 2021

New cases and hospitalizations have both been declining since February 1, but the death rate remains steady with three thousand Americans dying from COVID each day; there were 32,000 deaths in the past eleven days.

Vaccination rates have improved, with a daily average of 1.7 million people receiving a first or second dose leading to a steady increase in the number of vaccinations. In fact, President Biden spoke to the nation yesterday, announcing that his administration had contracted with vaccine producers for an additional two hundred million doses, and combined with what was previously secured, it is enough to vaccinate three hundred million Americans by the end of July.

A year into the pandemic, the CDC has issued guidelines for schools to open using a science-based approach, including common-sense mitigation efforts and a color-coded classification based on the number of cases per 100,000. This is the same plan the state of Oregon used to determine that the children in Wallowa County can attend in-person classes but the children in Portland must continue remote learning.

In Massachusetts, a new plan to help seniors navigate the vaccination system allowed their caregivers to also receive vaccines, leading to cash offerings from young adults who wanted to pose as "companions." More line-jumping.

In the Senate impeachment trial of the ex-president, the prosecution presented its case for insurrection over two days of compelling testimony including texts, speeches, chat room posts, phone videos and photos and security footage taken during the insurrection. The trial presents yet another opportunity for those Republican Senators who are afraid of the ex-president and his "base" to finally do the right thing. The soul of the nation is at stake; history will remember.

FEBRUARY 13, 2021

Despite an exceptionally stunning case presented by the House managers, the ex-president was acquitted for the second time by a vote of 57 to 43 which is a few votes short of the two-thirds super-majority required to convict. The Senate majority leader, Mitch McConnell—now the minority leader—voted to acquit due to a "lack of jurisdiction," meaning since the coup leader is no longer president, the Senate cannot impeach him, which is circular thinking that most constitutional scholars have publicly and loudly dismissed.

We all remember that Senate Leader McConnell was the one who delayed the Senate trial until after the inauguration so his Republican caucus could use this defense. There are forty-three cowards currently in the Senate who have cast another vote for dictatorship.

Ironically, the entire Senate gave Officer Goodman of the Capitol Hill police a standing ovation and the Medal of Honor for protecting those same Senators during the insurrection. We saw dramatic video footage of him leading the rioters away from the Senate doors, of re-directing a Senator who was heading into danger, of helping evacuate the Senate chambers. He was highly praised for protecting the Senate, but of course the Senate did not protect us from the man who started it all—who summoned and incited and unleashed the mob because he lost an election.

Due to the insurrection, our nation's capital still looks like a war zone with razor wire circling the grounds and National Guard troops on patrol. So much for the peaceful transfer of power...the bedrock of our democracy. By the time my grandchildren read this journal, there will have been another four presidential elections. Let's hope this is an object lesson not easily forgotten; let's hope every future generation is required to study this exceptional betrayal by Republican leaders.

FEBRUARY 14, 2021

	Cases	Deaths	Daily new	Daily deaths
World:	108,817,000	2,400,000	277,853	6,123
US:	27,600,000	485,800	72,164	1,366

There is a common frog fable that describes human behavior so well it is used to explain the inexplicable and it goes like this: If you drop a frog in boiling water, it will jump out immediately, but if you drop the frog in warm water and turn up the heat it will boil to death.

Now that the US is down to ONLY 100,000 new cases per day, and under 100,000 hospitalization, and less than 4,000 daily deaths, some governors have decided to relax or even end restrictions—including mask mandates—and open schools and restaurants and bars. They have a new sense of security from the post-surge drop in numbers and the initial rollout of vaccines, but ending mitigation efforts while the variant is spreading will entice the sleepy frog to a slow death.

In New Zealand, a three-day lockdown has been ordered after three people in one family reported unexplained infections. This is the frog-dropped-in-boiling-water part of our scenario. The government answers every rise in temperature with a rapid response and has been exceedingly successful: There have been 2,300 cases and twenty-five deaths in New Zealand during the entire pandemic. They stop and jump when cases are reported and as a result, the country is open for business most of the time, all their children are in school, and loved ones do not die alone in crowded hospitals.

The UK variant has now been found in eighty-two countries and is spreading so fast in the US that variant cases double every ten days. Researchers now suspect an increase in viral load causes a 35-45% increase in transmission and warn that this variant will be the dominant strain in the US by March.

While some in the US bathe in the warmth of lower numbers and vaccines, the new variant is quietly turning up the heat.

February 16, 2021

Extreme cold not seen in decades has shut down much of the central US. Dangerous roads have caused accidents and traffic jams, and high demand for electricity left millions of people in Texas without power during the coldest three nights in memory. Water lines have burst from the freezing cold, so people use snow to flush toilets.

Texas, one of the richest states in the union due to the oil industry, maintains an independent energy grid to avoid the cost of cold-weather precautions the federal government requires. Their grid is now failing due to freezing temperatures, and because they are not connected to the national energy network, they cannot import help from neighboring states.

Currently, there are rolling blackouts designed to avoid a catastrophic cascading grid failure but the blackouts have lasted three days already. Water pipes are still bursting, and they have issued a "boil water" warning for all of Houston.

Of course, millions have no electricity and no water so there is nothing to boil and no way to boil it. Grocery shelves are empty, so people are waiting in long lines in frigid weather out of desperation for food. There are pictures of homes flooded and icicles hanging from ceiling fans. People are freezing and angry and dozens have already died from the storm. It may be hard for people to understand that a warming arctic sends frigid air south, but that is happening—the result of global warming. The state of Texas is dependent on profits from refining fossil fuel so global warming is considered a hoax for political and economic reasons.

There were also deadly tornadoes in North Carolina and ice storms in Austin—and here in the Pacific Northwest—that sent cracked limbs crashing into power lines. Nearly 73% of the continental US is covered in cold and snow and there is more extreme weather on the way. A new record was set in Hastings, Nebraska with a temperature of thirty below zero, and Oklahoma reported a temperature of minus 14, the coldest morning since 1899. A few unlucky families forgot about carbon monoxide poisoning and were found "unresponsive" after huddling together to stay warm in cars that were still idling inside the garage.

People can deny climate change all they want but beliefs do not change facts. And the governor of Texas can blame windmills for the grid failure, but the truth is that Texas politicians have buried their proverbial heads in the sand—in oil wells—for a hundred years, and for this the people of Texas now shiver and freeze, suffering so others can profit.

FEBRUARY 17, 2021

Daily cases of new COVID infections have been under 100,000 for a week, raising hope that our winter surge is waning. In addition, the death rate and hospitalization numbers are steadily falling. More than 48 million doses of the vaccine have been administered reaching 12% of the population in the US.

Recent testing shows the Pfizer and Moderna vaccines are both highly effective against the UK variant and somewhat effective against the South African variant; both companies plan to develop boosters to upgrade protection against future variants. President Biden still promises there will be enough vaccine by the end of July to provide two shots to everyone in the US who wants them—600 million doses for 300 million adults. They are currently testing the safety of the vaccine for children.

The CDC announced that people who are fully vaccinated with two doses do not have to quarantine if exposed to the virus. And in more good news, Dr. Fauci echoed President Biden's promise that things will be nearly normal by Christmas this year.

The winter storms have slowed down the delivery of vaccines, so I may not receive a first dose on March 1st, but I am still hopeful. Keith is fully vaccinated, being two weeks out from his second shot on February 4th.

Unfortunately, there are still 130 countries that have not seen a single dose of vaccine. We can only hope that the US will continue to ramp up supply so everyone in the world can be vaccinated. Only herd immunity on a global scale will finally end the crisis.

FEBRUARY 19, 2021

The pandemic has been with us for a year and has changed our nation more than we know. So, what has changed? To start, our understanding of inequality.

When a pandemic disproportionately affects the bottom two-thirds of the population—when the poor are exposed more often and experience more illness—the stark reality of our inequality is quantified daily in death counts and food lines.

For decades we divided ourselves into "white collar" and "blue collar" and were comfortable with this distinction because we believed we could freely choose; those who enjoyed school went to school and those who wanted to work with their hands did so and everyone had a shot at the American dream.

But we ignored the privilege involved—the legacy, the resources, the expectations—and convinced ourselves that getting ahead was the result of hard work. We ignored the fact that the safety net for those who worked with their hands—the unions that ensured a living wage and benefits—was deliberately dismantled during the past fifty years along with the middle class.

As a result, white-collar workers became "elites" and blue-collar workers became disgruntled because the standard of living their parents enjoyed was now beyond their reach. It was easy to blame others—the minorities and immigrants who worked the low-wage jobs no one else wanted—and politicians successfully campaigned on blame.

Another telling story about inequality in America, the story the pandemic and the Trump presidency so clearly highlights, is the systematic oppression of minorities through instruments of racism, institutional barriers so thoroughly integrated into society, most of us have been blind to both the cause and the result: White privilege.

We have allowed voter suppression and educational disparity and financial barriers to draw sharp lines around neighborhoods, and then we trained men who are comfortable with violence to enforce these unspoken racial rules. Over time we integrated the prejudices of our forefathers so fully that they rise and fall like a faint heartbeat within us, undetected and silently tolerated until an enforcer kneels on a neck for nine minutes and twenty-nine seconds, killing in broad daylight.

White privilege is the opposite of racial justice and poverty is the result, a weakness the virus exploits. Without adequate healthcare and income—without a universal safety net—minorities suffer and die at a much higher rate.

We wonder how this pandemic year has changed Americans. For some of us, it has clearly exposed inequality and the racism it protects. For others—for the racists and misogynists living among us—they no longer feel the need to hide.

FEBRUARY 22, 2021

Today we reached a heartbreaking milestone: 28 million recorded cases in the US and 500,000 deaths from COVID in the past year, the highest number of deaths anywhere in the world. Exactly one year ago there were thirty-five cases and no deaths in the US.

The consequences are dire: Most of us have been isolating in our homes for a year, most of our children are not in classrooms or boardrooms, most small-business owners have financial challenges, and many will never open their doors again. At least eighteen million people are still unemployed, considered low due to the additional millions—mostly women—who have left the work force permanently due to a lack of childcare. The unofficial unemployment rate is 10%.

Dr. Fauci was quoted as saying that political divisions are responsible for the high death rate in the US, meaning the ex-president made the pandemic a political issue and his supporters refused to follow mitigation efforts and occasionally attacked those who did. Studies show he lost the election because of his failed pandemic response.

President Biden lined the outside staircase of the White House with five hundred candles, each representing a thousand loved ones who died of COVID in the past year. The president spoke of extraordinary people and observed a moment of silence with his wife, and with the vice president and her husband, the second gentleman.

He reminded us that more Americans have died of COVID in the past twelve months than from all the combat deaths during all the years of war in which our soldiers fought and died. He was solemn and sincere when he said we needed to grieve as a nation, to recognize the heartbreaking loss of life so many are facing every day.

One wonders if we might reach or even surpass the death rate from the 1918 Spanish flu—655,000 US dead—when they also ignored the pandemic for political reasons AND had no antivirals or antibiotics or vaccines to stop the spread or treat the illness.

We must do better than a century ago. How can we not do better?

FEBRUARY 25, 2021

The United States spent $782 billion on the military in 2020, a sum greater than the next seven nations combined. China was the nearest competitor with much less than half our spending ($261 billion), with India at $71 billion, and Russia—our great enemy—with just $65 billion in a year.

We are told this level of spending is required to keep us safe from aggressors and to maintain a position of leadership in the world. This extraordinary spending is not a surprise when you consider the US maintains nearly eight hundred bases in seventy countries staffed by three million uniformed souls who serve in one of our seven branches of the military. Exploring the reasons why we maintain this military empire is a question best left for another day.

But it was not an invading army that closed our borders, and it was not our robust military that countered the threat to our economy and entire social structure; not even $782 billion in military spending could protect our quality of life in 2020. Our robust war machine is designed for conventional threats—as a defense to secure borders and political ideology and economic dominance, and an offense to keep other nations at bay.

Eisenhower warned us about the "military industrial complex" after World War II, a gigantic profit center not easily dismantled. Seventy-five years later, we still spend hundreds of billions of dollars to protect the nation and are brought to our knees by a microscopic virus. Something needs to change.

The modern threats to our way of life are global and not subject to physical borders: a changing climate, diminished natural resources, economic inequality...threats that all the military hardware and all the forces in uniform cannot address without a response rooted in science.

The virus caught us unprepared because science became a political issue, a tug of war between profit and progress. We know from history that when profits are threatened, progress is stalled and the common good is lost for a time.

We also know that when we face a challenge and partner with science miracles happen...like a vaccine developed in less than a year using innovative technology that will provide new ways to fight deadly diseases in the future.

Here is an idea: Instead of gender-based birthday gifts—toy guns and Barbie dolls—we might want to give our children real microscopes and chemistry sets and invest as early as possible in the quality of mind needed to solve modern problems.

FEBRUARY 26, 2021

	CASES	DEATHS	DAILY NEW	DAILY DEATHS
WORLD:	113,416,000	2,516,000	414,192	9,798
US:	28,500,000	511,619	78,262	2,266

A giant golden idol rolled across the stage at the annual Conservative Political Action Conference (CPAC) to honor Donald Trump, a man who was impeached twice, who tore immigrant children from the arms of parents, who inspired an insurrection against Congress, who lost the House and the Senate and the presidency by seven million votes, who threatens democracy with his every lie; a golden idol made real by mixing ignorance with a hunger for power and a made-up victory in the midst of defeat...because the repeating of a lie apparently makes it so.

Sanity requires a special effort now: The Big Lie of a stolen election has become the dominant Republican narrative, and a defeated and disgraced con man still leads this cult from the comfort of his gilded golf club in Florida.

Part Five: Hope and Hysteria

March 1—July 15, 2021

MARCH 1, 2021

The virus is an early retrograde mutation of an organism that can only reproduce after attaching to—and using—cell proteins, unlike bacteria that can reproduce independent of a host. Bacteria are free-living cells that can reproduce inside or outside a body, while viruses are a collection of molecules that need a host to survive. Viruses are much smaller than bacteria cells and can survive extreme temperatures in a non-living state. Once they attach to a protein in the living host, they can reproduce at will and mutate when needed to survive immune system defenses.

Antibodies are the best defense, but the virus can alter cell proteins which will inhibit the attachment of antibodies and create a new variation of itself that is more dangerous than the original—more transmissible and sometimes more lethal.

We now have vaccines that are very effective against the original virus and somewhat effective against the early variants. We may need a COVID booster every year to address the mutations of this virus while it tries to survive against vaccines and herd immunity.

This week Johnson & Johnson began shipping doses of their new vaccine after receiving approval from the FDA. This one-dose vaccine is around 72% effective in preventing infection and highly effective in limiting severe illness. It can be shipped easily since it needs no refrigeration. The company expects to have twenty million doses in arms by the end of March and have announced a production partnership with Merck that will provide enough vaccine for every American by the end of May—two months earlier than previously expected.

Globally, there are forty vaccines in Phase 1 human trials, twenty-seven vaccines in Phase 2 trials, twenty in Phase 3 mass trials, with six approved for emergency use. Vaccine diplomacy between nations has created unusual alliances as governments scramble to acquire enough doses to vaccinate their people. Very few nations have more than 12% of their citizens vaccinated so far. It will take a year or more to vaccinate the entire world against COVID.

I have been scheduled for my first dose on March 5 at 9:45 at Cloverleaf Hall in Enterprise, along with my brother and his wife. We are going to celebrate this happy event together on Friday afternoon. Rachel and Kevin and Michael are still waiting, but pregnant women are next in line in Colorado so Rachel should be vaccinated soon. Keith had his first haircut in fourteen months.

MARCH 5TH, 2021

Today was vaccination day for my brother and my sister-in-law and me. We moved through a smooth process with our neighbors over sixty-five and felt relief and joy in Cloverleaf Hall while we greeted masked friends from a distance for the first time in a year.

Vaccination sites are in full swing throughout America—in small community centers and large stadiums and convention centers. Yankee stadium will vaccinate New Yorkers 24/7 until everyone who wants a shot has received one. The National Guard is manning four hundred centers across the nation.

While I recovered from my shot—slight headache, fatigue, and muscle aches—I watched *I am Legend*, a movie about a virus gone wrong starring Will Smith. Virologists thought they had manipulated a virus to cure cancer, but due to mutations, it killed 90% of humanity outright and turned 9% into blood-thirsty zombies who then fed on the one percent who were immune. Smith's character eventually discovered a cure but sacrificed himself to ensure the vaccine reached the immune who were barricaded together, thus saving humanity.

The anti-vaxxers find confirmation in this movie along with the online conspiracy theories that claim the vaccine changes DNA, that the government delivers tracking devises via the vaccine, that there is a risk of life-changing side-effects. *I am Legend* fictionalized the worst-case scenario of a vaccine not fully tested or controlled, but the current science of vaccines has evolved at the fastest pace in history due to the global effort to stop this virus. Humanity will benefit.

The Detroit mayor is under fire for rejecting the Johnson & Johnson vaccine saying they had enough of the first two vaccines; the optics are bad when the effort to vaccinate everyone depends on this simpler vaccine that uses traditional flu technology. Regardless of being slightly less effective, this one dose vaccine did prevent severe illness and hospitalizations and deaths in the trials…a valuable tool in the arsenal.

Fear of the vaccine is our enemy now.

MARCH 7, 2021

There are now ten different vaccines being distributed in the world with varied success. Israel is the vaccination leader with 55% of the population vaccinated and the UK is at 32% although they are administering only the first dose of a two-dose vaccine. The US vaccination rate is 16%.

The overall vaccination rate in North America is 14.9%; Europe is 8.8%; South America is 3.7%; Asia is 2.3%; Africa 0.3%. So far, only 312 million doses of the vaccine have been administered in a world with over eight billion souls.

While many areas of the world are reporting a significant decline in cases and deaths, Brazil is still a mess, with a deadly variant reinfecting people who were previously sick but recovered, and an incompetent president who told the Brazilian people to stop whining. The hospitals are nearly 100% full and there is no oxygen, so now some practice "terminal sedation," which means they administer enough morphine to put people to sleep while they die.

Only 4% of the population in Brazil has been vaccinated and several new variants have been discovered in areas where few mitigation strategies are in place. Scientists say the infection rate in Brazil led to new variants and the country is a ticking bomb.

In fact, the new variants from Brazil are a threat to the 90% of the world that has not yet been vaccinated. New hotspots on top of old hotspots are being reported and much of the world has remained at some level of lockdown... but not all. You can still travel to Brazil if you choose.

In Oregon, a virus sample was discovered with the UK variant and the South American variant combined, the first of its kind, which has the scientists baffled. The subject did not travel out of state, so it was a unique mutation with community spread. We are hoping for a failed mutation.

In Idaho—our neighbor to the east—a hundred far-right activists staged an anti-mask protest on the steps of the state capitol yesterday and made the national news when they encouraged small children to throw their masks into the flames. They chanted "freedom" and pumped fists in the air for the camera. As political scientist Ian Bremmer said: "Ritualized mask burning in Boise wins this week's award for acts of symbolic stupidity." They have my vote.

MARCH 9, 2021

62,000,000 vaccines administered in the US

Keith had double knee replacement surgery yesterday in Vancouver, Washington. It felt strange to be driving in a big city, picking up food at restaurants, staying in a hotel, walking into public buildings…always with a mask, as quickly as possible. Without time to build antibodies, I am still unprotected and very cautious.

The $1.9 trillion American Rescue package was passed by the House and the Senate, and President Biden will sign it into law this week. According to Bernie Sanders, an independent Vermont senator, it is the "most significant legislation for working people passed in twenty-five years," which is high praise coming from the most vocal progressive in the Senate. Not a single Republican voted for the American Rescue bill, citing the high cost, even though the 2017 Trump tax cut had a similar price tag and mainly benefited corporations and the wealthiest one-percent of the public.

Economic stimulus is critical now. During the past year, poverty has been a leading factor in COVID hospitalizations and deaths due to crowded living quarters, poor healthcare, and low-quality food. And many of those in poverty have service jobs and are designated essential workers—delivery drivers and grocery store clerks, workers in meat-packing plants, personal-care assistants—working for minimum wage with no safety net when they fall sick and lose jobs. The death rate for Latino men is seven times higher than for White men due to more job exposure and less access to healthcare.

There are still long lines at food banks, and millions of unemployed Americans have mounting debt from the housing crisis. The new stimulus package is designed to address significant debt, food scarcity, education deficits, and small-business bankruptcy—a few of the targeted resources included in the package. Economists say those in the bottom 20% of the economy will find their standard of living raised by 20% due to stimulus spending. Some are calling the package "Biden's New Deal."

A study published today by Johns Hopkins reported that in states led by Republican governors the infection and death rates were 1.8 times higher during the second half of 2020 than in states led by Democratic governors due to the political rhetoric from party leaders—nearly two times more infection and death.

It is not a surprise. The same people who supported the Republican president are the ones who burned their masks and now refuse to get vaccinated—41% of all Republicans and 49% of Republican men have said they do not plan to get a shot. It would have helped if the outgoing president had joined the past presidents in advocating for vaccination, but Trump and his wife received shots in secret before leaving the White House in disgrace and have said nothing about the benefits of vaccination to their base.

In other news, the FBI announced they have made 320 arrests in the Capitol insurrection investigation and expect to make a hundred more. They have access to 15,000 digital images, have issued nine hundred search warrants in fifty states, have fielded 210,000 hotline tips, and collected 1,600 witness statements. They are building a case for an insurrection conspiracy that reaches all the way to the previous White House administration.

MARCH 11, 2021

Today marks the one-year anniversary of the announcement by the WHO that Coronavirus was a global pandemic—an epidemic that reached every continent and every country. In January 2020 we were told it was not airborne, in February that it was under control, and by March we realized delayed warnings allowed travelers to spread the disease around the world—first in Asia, then to Europe and the Americas, and finally Africa. By the time the WHO warned us on March 11, 2020, it was too late.

Today also marks the one-year anniversary of this journal, a project that has filled my time while isolating at home; a writing project that has covered lockdowns and protests, hurricanes and wildfires and plagues of locust, race riots and insurrection, infection and death rates, loneliness and grief.

To mark the pandemic anniversary, President Biden made his first address to the nation with news of progress against the virus and a warning not to let down our guard. As a candidate he promised that controlling the pandemic would be his first priority and so far, he has kept his word.

President Biden has approved a stimulus bill, has secured a robust supply chain for vaccine materials, has signed contracts with pharmaceutical companies to ramp up vaccine production, and promised enough vaccine by May 1 to offer a shot to every US adult.

It is important to reflect on the past year by recognizing the loss caused by COVID and the progress we have made. Most children have not been in school since last March, so parents working from home have also become educators—suddenly isolated and ill-prepared for a double workload. The children suffered without personal contact with friends. They also missed the after-school activities—no sports, music, dance, art—which means they also had no in-person contact with non-parental adults…no coaches or mentors or teachers. The good news is that 60% of schools will reopen by the end of this month, and there is talk of summer school to make up for lost time.

And for those of us retired there has been no travel, no theater, no movies, no concerts, no restaurant dining, no museums, no bustling cities, no visits with our elderly beloved, no service projects. None. For a year. But the good news is that we can travel again this summer with very little risk, at least domestically.

With more than half a million deaths, a third of us have lost a loved one from COVID in the past year; with nearly thirty million infections recorded in the US, all of us know someone who was sick with the virus. The "long-haulers" are still sick a year later; a new medical specialty will track this disease for decades to come. We have discovered new virus treatments and vaccine technology to use against future pandemics.

Although two-thirds of the deaths in the US occurred among the elderly last year, the death rate in nursing homes is down 90% due to early vaccinations; most homes are now open to visitors. Imagine elderly loved ones having no personal contact for the entire year—no daughters or sons or grandchildren to hug. They can finally visit face-to-face with family again.

And, of course, we are not out of the woods yet: The airports set a record on Friday with the most travelers in over a year; Florida beaches are crowded with college students on spring break; states are ending mitigation efforts just as variants are spreading; we still have a thousand or two dying every day from the virus.

But the race between the variants and the vaccines seems to be moving in our favor and the country with the worst pandemic response is now the nation with the most vaccine; one in five Americans have been vaccinated.

MARCH 15, 2021

The streets of Italy are empty again. Last March they were the first country in Europe to lock down—with a high virus rate and overwhelming death—and they are locked down again due to a third wave of infection caused by the UK variant.

A year ago, the image of Italians gathered on apartment balconies in the early evening—to greet each other and sing to healthcare workers—was one of the most iconic images of the early pandemic along with an empty St. Peter's Square and deserted city streets.

These images shocked us…but that was before we saw long lines of sick patients in New York City and hospital tents in Central Park and refrigerated trucks parked outside city morgues; before the virus spread across continents and oceans and countries and states and cities and neighborhoods and into our homes; before every country in the world was infected.

The UK variant is now raging in Europe and there are indications of another, bigger wave. Each European country has a unique mitigation strategy that may include curfews, lockdowns, limits on gatherings, restaurant closures, shopping appointments, or closed borders so it is a challenge to track the European Union but there are increasing restrictions in every country due to the surge from variants.

Like the rest of the world, Europe is in a race between variants and vaccinations. And in most countries, vaccines are in limited supply due to material shortages and factory delays, problems the US has finally solved.

In addition, anti-vaccine sentiments are causing hesitation to receive shots among those who fear vaccines in general due to the vaccination conspiracy theory that originated in England decades ago. And now, an unproven link between the AstraZeneca vaccine and blood clots was proof enough for nine countries in the European Union to suspend its use pending investigation, further limiting supply on the eve of an infection wave. Europe is in a race and one of their shoes just fell off.

India is facing their second wave. Initially, the virus was slow to spread during the first wave due to low infection rates in a nation with a young and healthy population. But when they suddenly entered lockdown in the fall, there was concern that their mobile workforce would return to villages and spread the virus. A strong mitigation effort helped control the first wave which peaked in September 2020 and showed steady improvement until early last month.

A second wave is hitting the cities, with some areas of India experiencing a 150% increase in infection rates. The vaccination rollout has not been smooth since the Modi government used an internet-based appointment system and only 50% of Indians have access to a computer or phone. In addition, vaccine hesitancy is fueled by misinformation flowing first on the Internet and then spreading like wildfire through the dense neighborhoods they call "slums" in megacities that are home to twenty million souls.

MARCH 17, 2021

	CASES	DEATHS	DAILY NEW	DAILY DEATHS
WORLD:	121,298,800	2,281,200	535,358	10,227
US:	29,632,000	537,649	58,856	1,177

A year ago, American passengers on a COVID-infected cruise ship were allowed to disembark in Florida without a test, walk through a crowded seaport, and return to their states and neighborhoods, bringing the virus with them.

And when the US suddenly "closed" borders to travelers from China and Europe, Americans living abroad rushed to re-enter the US and were allowed to leave the airports without tests because there were no tests. The CDC initially sent flawed tests to states and then rejected accurate tests from independent labs because they had no protocol in place for approval. The CDC was totally unprepared and quickly overwhelmed.

Yesterday, three women from a neighboring town who planned to fly to Belize tested positive for the virus a few days before departure and were blocked by the airline even after a second test was negative. After review, it was determined that the three were on the tail end of an asymptomatic infection that cleared before the second test. But they had no time to take a third test, which is required to remove the block, and had to cancel the trip.

What a difference a year makes in a pandemic. If we had been able to test last March when the COVID virus first arrived on planes and boats, we might have skipped the spring wave and the summer wave and the winter holiday wave...and the second spring wave currently brewing.

Hannah celebrated her 28th birthday yesterday but instead of going to bars in downtown Portland with friends like she did at the beginning of the pandemic in 2020, she went to a surprise party thrown by a few medical school classmates who are all fully vaccinated. It was a good reminder that after a year of isolation and heartache, we can now gather a few at a time.

MARCH 18, 2021

100,000,000 vaccine doses administered in the US

A *Lancet* magazine article in September 2020 compared three genetically similar viruses found this century for transmissibility and lethality.

The Sars-CoV-1 virus appeared in 2002 with 8,098 cases worldwide and 774 deaths (a 14% lethality). The MERS virus was detected in 2012 with 2,494 cases and 858 deaths due to a high fatality rate (34%).

The Sars-Cov-2 (COVID-19) virus appeared in October 2019 and has infected nearly 122 million people worldwide and killed 2.7 million so far due to a high transmissibility rate in addition to asymptomatic infections. Fatality rates range from under 1% for children to over 15% for the elderly.

The first SARS virus had a transmission rate (R0) of two (two new infections for every one already infected) with a slow development of virus load so the long incubation allowed more days for contact tracing and quarantine; there appeared to be no asymptomatic transmission. The second SARS virus (COVID-19) has a transmission rate of 2.5 and an incubation for contagion of six days on average. Nearly half the people infected had no symptoms when they infected others, so the new virus spread like wildfire...often without coughs or fever or pain.

There have been many theories about how this virus originated and spread: that it was developed by some military group and deliberately released, or that it was stored in a substandard scientific facility and walked out on someone's shoe.

The most logical theory is that an unfortunate contact with a sick animal infected a human host with a new virus and it spread when they went shopping in a crowded animal market in Wuhan, China a few days later.

Any number of small incidental changes in the chain of contact could have eliminated the threat of a global pandemic; many new viruses never find lethal expression. But in this case the stars were aligned: successful contact, asymptomatic infection, crowded conditions, and airborne transmission all combined to make this virus successfully deadly.

The ex-president built his base on White grievance so he named SARS-CoV-2 the "China Virus" and repeated this racial dog whistle to adoring crowds. Racist attacks on Asian Americans increased exponentially in 2020, and just today a 21-year-old gunman opened fire at three different day spas in Atlanta, killing eight people including six young Korean women.

Words have even greater consequences in the age of social media since anger can fester in a sick mind, spread with a few strokes on a keyboard, and infect the public square with deadly results…just like a virus.

MARCH 22, 2021

Today we dismantled Pandemic Porch. The cafe lights were gathered and piled; the heavy tarps were separated from the supporting steel rods and folded for storage. The stand-up heater will remain for cold spring nights on the porch with our friends now that we are all vaccinated. For the past year, those in our retired friend group were able to isolate at home and wait patiently for the vaccine. We were fortunate and we survived.

The young adults have run out of patience. Miami Beach has been overrun with students on spring break and their pent-up passions have led to dangerous behavior. In addition to packed crowds and curfew violations, there have been fights with police leading to hundreds of arrests and at least one deadly sexual assault that we know of so far.

There was another mass shooting by a 21-year-old in Colorado last night, and I can't help but wonder if the stress of the previous year is exploding inside those without the strength to emerge healthy from lockdown; those with pent-up rage from isolation who are re-entering a world that is both fragile and unfriendly. Murder rates are on the rise.

Suicides are also on the rise, another indication of how the virus feeds on weakness. We are hungry by design—for love, friendship, accomplishment—and the isolation of the past year has compounded that hunger in those who struggle to find emotional support.

Hopefully, we are near the end. Nearly 25% of Americans have had at least one shot, and we may have some herd immunity by late summer. We will all be emerging from isolation during the next few months and none of us will be whole, not yet, but we do have hope—and a profound need for kindness.

MARCH 24, 2021

The European Union continues to botch the vaccine rollout. They managed to export more vaccine than they distributed to their twenty-seven member nations due to a less aggressive posture to secure vaccine and a lack of regulation for exporting the vaccine they produced. A recently discovered stash of 29 million doses of the AstraZeneca vaccine in Italy gives rise to speculation that producers were looking for a more favorable market outside the European Union.

Britain has been aggressively importing from the EU even though they also produced vaccines locally. As a result, Britain has vaccinated nearly 43% of their population while Germany, Italy, Spain, and France have each vaccinated less than 10%.

These distribution problems are now referred to as vaccine nationalism, the flip side of vaccine diplomacy. A few nations hoard supply while other nations use the promise of vaccine to secure new allies. The US has been on the hoarder side of the coin until recently. We finally agreed to "loan" AstraZeneca doses to Canada and Mexico after international criticism and a dawning realization that herd immunity transcends borders.

In other places, vaccine hesitancy is a bigger problem. In Hong Kong, only 39% of residents are willing to take the vaccine due to a lack of trust in the Chinese government who tried to reassert control of the country last year. In the Middle East, less than 50% of health care workers trust the vaccine since all doses are imported.

We also have rising vaccine hesitancy here in the US due to the far right adopting a "Stop the vaccine" platform after failing to "Stop the steal." In addition, the Russian propaganda machine provides ample misinformation online in a campaign designed to protect their own global vaccine profits while vexing the American people.

Another unique vaccination problem is line-skipping and the havoc it creates among friends. Vaccination centers take everyone at their word, so it is easy for someone to claim an "underlying conditions" and skip ahead of their assigned place. Cheaters do not realize how shallow their cheating looks on social media when they celebrate vaccination; they are clueless when friends express strong feelings about cheating because they are worried for their own parents and grandparents.

But these are rich nation problems. Brazil, with a 5.8% vaccination rate and a raging variant, reported a record of 3,251 deaths yesterday; they have lost control of the pandemic. India, with only 3.3% of the public vaccinated, reported 53,000 new infections, the highest number since the peak of their first wave in October.

Here is the real vaccine story: There are currently forty-three nations that will have almost everyone vaccinated within the year; there are 148 nations that will not be done for a year after that; there are still sixty-seven nations that have no vaccine—sixty-seven nations that have not vaccinated a single person.

MARCH 26, 2021

Four days ago, one of the largest container ships in the world, carrying 20,000 fully loaded steel boxes on a ship measuring a quarter mile long, was lodged sideways in the Suez Canal, due to heavy wind and human error, and still blocks the entire shipping lane.

There are hundreds of ships and barges stuck in front and behind the *Ever Given,* with billions of dollars of cargo just sitting and waiting to reach European ports; there are hundreds more ships taking the long way around the Horn of Africa to avoid the blocked canal, which requires an extra week of sailing and additional fuel. The entire global supply chain has been affected by the calamity. Once the canal is cleared, thousands of ships will arrive in ports simultaneously and then wait again to unload.

This is a modern-day global supply chain problem caused by the digital marketplace. Manufacturers are now able to produce and ship goods on demand instead of trying to anticipate future sales and stockpile merchandise. There is rarely an emergency stash of needed supplies stored in a warehouse, something we learned from experience early in the pandemic; healthcare workers and anxious consumers waited weeks for protective gear and hand sanitizer...and toilet paper.

There is concern that Brazil is becoming a threat to the world. Following Trump's lead, the Brazilian president, Bolsonaro denied the risk of the pandemic throughout 2020 and denies it still in 2021. His attitude has been condemned worldwide but due to the new Brazilian variant, his indifference has now become an even greater threat at home with soaring infections among the younger population, a collapsing healthcare system across the nation, and thousands of deaths per day—a perfect environment for new variants to find purchase and spread.

Political indifference in Brazil can infect the whole world. A second pandemic could arise from the first, a more transmissible and lethal "variant of a variant" that will require new mitigation efforts and new vaccines. As goes the part in Brazil, so goes the whole world.

MARCH 29, 2021

There are 40,000 deaths by firearms each year in the US; thousands of children have been shot and killed in the past twenty years because loaded guns were left lying around. Americans make up just over five percent of the global population but own 42% of all the guns in the world—400 million guns in the US.

Most Americans are appalled by these statistics and wonder why we cannot enact common-sense gun laws. How did the second amendment's guarantee of a "well-armed militia" for defense of a new country morph into a personal right for every adult to own a semi-automatic weapon capable of firing hundreds of rounds a minute?

Once again, we see that personal freedom without social responsibility is the flag of false liberty. When White nationalists with semi-automatic weapons took over the Michigan statehouse in the name of personal freedom, we had an object lesson in false liberty. When the Proud Boys and the Oath Keepers planned and executed an insurrection aimed at the heart of our democracy on January 6th, we witnessed the destruction caused by false liberty when used as a weapon by self-serving politicians.

The global pandemic has required suffocating limits on our personal freedom and for some it has been too difficult; they feel compelled to fight restrictions regardless of the public good. But what if we all carried semi-automatic weapons to make a point and stormed the public square to change the vote and ignored the virus and the science and the vaccine? What would happen then?

The virus would win and the people with guns would rule.

MARCH 31, 2021

	Cases	Deaths	Daily new	Daily deaths
World:	128,988,900	2,816,900	676,789	12,241
US:	30,485,200	551,636	68,162	1,138

Several one-year reviews of the pandemic—on the origin of the virus and the global leadership response—have been published or aired this week.

The WHO released its first report on the origin of the virus and fourteen nations immediately objected to the report due to claims that China caused a delay in the release of the report and refused to provide supporting data. Even with no conclusive findings, the team of seventeen international scientists said it was *likely to highly likely* that the virus spread from animal to human in a market, and *highly unlikely* that there was a laboratory accident although further research into this scenario was warranted due to the prevalence of several virology labs in Wuhan where the virus originated.

In a CNN special report, six members of the US COVID Task Force under the former president were interviewed to provide an "autopsy" of our failed response to the pandemic in 2020. Here are some of the highlights:

Dr. Fauci lamented that he would have been "horrified" in the beginning to know that over half a million Americans would die in 2020 from the virus. He also said it felt like a "gut punch" when the ex-president tweeted his encouragement to "liberate" various states and argued that we "open up for business" in the spring of 2020.

Dr. Birx said that after the first 100,000 deaths, the next 400,000 could have been prevented with an adequate response from the administration. She also reported that after the first shutdown in March, the ex-president warned her that the country would "never again shut down."

Several Health and Human Services officials in the Trump administration said there was no system in place to track supply chains for protective gear or testing components or ventilators. The ex-president's claims of "millions of tests" referred to individual components and wishful thinking.

All members interviewed said they had received death threats from the ex-president's supporters. (In response to the CNN special, Trump called the Task Force doctors "self-promoters" with bad instincts and faulty recommendations.)

In an opinion piece published in *The Washington Post*, Frida Ghitis documents the worst pandemic responses in the world over the past year. She compared the US, Brazil, Nicaragua, Mexico, Belarus, Turkmenistan, Cambodia, and Tanzania. These nations were all led by populist authoritarian leaders or dictators, all were men, all eventually contracted COVID, and all but one survived after receiving state-of-the-art medical care. And they all took a page from the US president's misinformation playbook and dismissed the pandemic in public.

Their pandemic responses included holding COVID parades, encouraging political rallies without masks, coughing and then shaking hands, refusing to count deaths, announcing the virus would magically "go away," advocating vodka and sauna as a cure, drinking bleach as a cure, banning masks, welcoming infected cruise ships, making it a crime to report COVID data, arresting activists, promoting ineffective anti-malarial treatments, calling it a little flu—the list goes on.

When all is said and done, it was the ex- president of the US who won the race, who caused the most death, prolonged the greatest suffering, shocked the world most often with his ignorant and seemingly intentional lack of leadership during the pandemic. So yes, he did make America "great" again.

On a positive note, twenty-four world leaders have formally signaled interest in developing a Global Pandemic Treaty to help us better prepare for the next viral threat. It is still early and the big players have yet to sign on, but there is hope that our pandemic response will be coordinated at a global level next time.

APRIL 2, 2021

Today was the second "vaccination day" for me and my brother and his wife, so after strolling into Cloverleaf Hall and getting our shot without a wait, we laminated the vaccination cards and then played dominoes in the sunshine, celebrating.

We were offered the Moderna shot and were thankful they were not offering AstraZeneca in the US since the controversy surrounding the vaccine developed at Oxford University continues. Recently we learned the AZ vaccine is 90% *ineffective* against the South African variant, B.1351.

There are six additional vaccines in Phase 3 trials which will bring the number available to ten if they are all approved by the FDA. We may be able to match a vaccine (or a booster) to the variants and find an effective response, but we are still in a race between the variants and the vaccines along with the rest of the world—the timeline for success is not yet certain.

Those of us in Oregon now have our second vaccines while Michael and Rachel and Kevin in Colorado are a week from their first. President Biden promised that all adults will be eligible by May 1, and he is right on target.

APRIL 4, 2021

For the past week the world has been watching the trial of a White police officer who responded to a call about a fake $20 bill by handcuffing a Black man, placing him face down on the asphalt, and digging his knee into the man's neck for nine minutes and twenty-nine seconds, killing him slowly while a crowd gathered and pleaded for his life. The entire world watched as the officer ignored the crowd, put his hands in his pockets and continued to suffocate the man with his knee. A paramedic had to literally pull the officer away from the suspect who had been unresponsive for nearly three minutes.

It was one year ago, on May 25 in Minneapolis, when the nation witnessed the murder of this unarmed Black man, George Floyd, by a White police officer, Derek Chauvin. Since that day there have been protests and rallies in nearly every city, discussions about race in every newspaper, debates on every news program...and likely at every dinner table.

It is a rare thing for a White officer to be found guilty of murdering a Black man, so the nation is holding its breath. Is it possible a jury will decide lethal aggression by a White police officer against a handcuffed Black suspect is acceptable?

Police violence against Black protesters was well documented last summer after George Floyd's death, but when White protesters stormed the capitol on January 6, the police response was muted; the few police on duty that day had no weapons, no backup, no orders to secure the perimeter even though the threat was known. The angry and mostly White mob was able to beat their way into the capitol, cause injury and death and destruction, and then return home for dinner. Five people were killed but there were no arrests on January 6. None.

During the past year we have seen that justice is not blind; White justice is not the same as Black justice and this racial disparity was not improved by civil rights legislation during the late 1960's. In fact, after Congress required desegregation in schools, law enforcement started a "war on drugs" which resulted in an incarceration rate that is nearly ten times greater for Blacks than Whites even though drug use is essentially the same. Black men make up 34% of the male prison population but only 6% of the US population.

Rules often change to ensure White privilege. Six White male politicians in Georgia just signed into law a new set of voting rights behind closed doors in response to the unprecedented surge in Black votes last fall. These Republican lawmen cite the "Big Lie" of voter fraud to justify Black voter suppression even though every judge who reviewed the 2020 election has ruled there was no fraud.

There are 361 similar voting rights bills to "fight fraud' sponsored by Republicans leaders in forty-seven states who are still trying to pretend they won. Republicans realize they cannot win without suppressing minority votes. When Black voters go to the polls and are willing to wait in long lines, rain or shine, democracy wins.

We can only hope that justice finally wins this week as well, that murder is murder no matter who commits it.

APRIL 6, 2021

It is heartening to see US vaccination trends improving. More than four million doses were administered on Saturday alone, and most states can comply with President Biden's new promise to open all vaccination sites to anyone over the age of sixteen on April 19—in two weeks. The expected timeline for herd immunity in the US has moved back to mid-summer if all goes well...if either new variants or vaccine ignorance does not derail progress.

There are many evangelicals—the 40 million right-to-life supporters of the ex-president—who are hesitant to receive the vaccine due to misinformation regarding the origin of the vaccine (did they use fetal stem cells?) and a general anti-science bias that defines the evangelical belief system, starting with the age of the planet and ending with the definition of human life.

Hesitancy also exists among (mostly) Republican men who have downplayed the pandemic due to politics, using very fluid "facts" that negate the need for vaccination. A public information campaign may help convince people to get the vaccine, but restrictions on the unvaccinated may be the stronger incentive in the long run. Vaccination passports are the new cultural flashpoint for the misinformed; they boldly refuse to take the vaccine but want all the benefits of those who do. Counterfeit vaccination cards flow through an online black market.

We are still in a race with the variants and have seen a 20% rise in infections during the past two weeks. Now that most of those 65 and older have been vaccinated, younger people are more at risk and suffer more severe symptoms. While states continue removing restrictions—and the stadiums and bars and theaters fill with the young and the restless—the variants find fertile ground.

The availability of the vaccine in the US is attracting expats home in record numbers. While vaccination rates are stalled in the rest of the world, President Biden's promise that all adults over the age of sixteen can get a shot is calling many Americans home.

APRIL 7, 2021

A year ago, 81% of the global workforce lost wages due to closures forced by the emerging pandemic. All at once the world was unemployed, the restaurants and theaters and museums were closed, the public squares were emptied; this time last year, the world was holding its breath.

Imagine Manhattan and Paris and Tokyo and London with no pedestrians, no cars, no public transportation…no place for anyone to go. Today, performers are returning to the stage and baseball teams are starting the season with actual fans in the stands.

A year ago, we wiped down everything we touched including steering wheels, packages, door handles, and groceries, but today the CDC finally admitted there was a 1 in 10,000 chance that someone could get the virus from a surface. COVID is airborne, and we are infected by breathing aerosolized virus particles, large and small.

A year ago, Europe and the US were the world's hotspots, especially among the elderly in nursing homes where the death toll reached double digits. A year ago, the ex-president promised "the virus will be gone by Easter" and encouraged us to "fill up the churches on Easter Sunday."

Two months ago, the US led the world with a third of the cases and a quarter of the deaths every day. Today, Brazil had a record 4,200 deaths and India recorded 126,000 infections—currently the highest counts in the world.

Fear of a fourth wave in the US is due to the spread of variants, but nearly 25% of the adult population has had at least one vaccine (50% here in Wallowa County.) We are ahead in the race to vaccinate…but with virus variants still raging around the world, anything can happen.

April 15, 2021

	Cases	Deaths	Daily new	Daily deaths
World:	**139,077,000**	**2,986,000**	**817,025**	**13,277**
US:	**31,500,000**	**564,600**	**73,116**	**867**

When both business and politics use misinformation to gain profit and power, the true *ideals* of the common good have been replaced by the false *ideas* of personal freedom.

But a commitment to the common good is the only thing that can guarantee personal freedom, as the framers of our Constitution attempted to codify. Now, in our confusion, personal freedom means an unlimited right to possess lethal weapons and to spread a deadly virus and to vilify the very same diversity that allowed our nation to grow and prosper; personal freedom has become a retrograde motion, a return to tribalism just when we most need to invest in the common good.

Science will be our salvation since the destruction of our environment by an unlimited hunger for profit has unleashed hazards—viruses and climate volatility—that only science can solve. Science requires the right mind, not the right race or religion or creed; science leads to evolution while tribalism leads to entropy—a closed system that feeds on itself.

Without a global scientific effort and the goal of worldwide vaccination, we will not defeat this virus. And unless we defeat the virus—and the ones to follow—none of us will be free.

APRIL 22, 2021

200,000,000 doses of the vaccine administered in the US

Due to a 47% increase in COVID infections in the state of Oregon during the two weeks following spring break, we have cancelled our trip to the coast. The governor will soon move fifteen counties to the highest COVID alert status—Extreme Risk—and that means restaurants, spas, museums and art galleries will close again. We are right back where we started this winter during the third wave; the fourth wave is upon us. Even though 50% of adults have been vaccinated, the highly transmissible variants are winning.

We know the vaccines work. Israel has vaccinated over 60% of adults and had no deaths from COVID this weekend for the first time in a year. But there is too much false information leading to vaccination hesitancy in this country. Self-proclaimed evangelical "prophets" are still preaching against this scientific breakthrough (as usual) and the weak-minded who follow conspiracy sites have a dozen reasons not to get the shot including a lingering theory that Bill Gates has inserted a microchip in the serum so he can track us. Cell phones must be obsolete.

The entire world is still at risk from the variants. The virus has exploded across India in a second wave and their healthcare system is collapsing. Funeral pyres are burning in the crematorium parking lots because there are too many bodies to burn inside. The hospitals are full and have no oxygen; people waiting in line are dying before finding a bed. India's official COVID infection tally for the past several days continues to exceed global records—there have been 352,000 infections in the past 24 hours—and some fear this is a fraction of the actual spread; many people die in India without receiving any treatment and without being counted.

Two months ago, there were 10,000 cases recorded per day and India's leaders claimed they defeated the virus. Now this country of 1.3 billion people is living the nightmare we all feared would come. In the state of Kolkata, with 15 million residents, 50% of those tested are positive. Most countries have closed borders to travelers from India. After facing international criticism over vaccine nationalism, the US will now send excess supply to India.

In Brazil, there is concern that tens of millions are going hungry. The government has reduced the payments that kept the poor fed; this affects more than half the country. And still the president of Brazil uses cruel bravado to shame those who fear the virus and are hungry for food and desperate for vaccines.

APRIL 24, 2001

In Minnesota, the White police officer who killed George Floyd a year ago by kneeling on his neck for nine minutes was convicted of all murder charges by a Minneapolis jury. This was considered unusual because only two of every two thousand deaths by police are prosecuted in this country; it is unusual because White police violence against Black men has been an acceptable strategy for controlling the "thugs." Derek Chauvin will spend at least twenty years in prison.

Even so, there were six questionable police killings of Black men and teenagers in the 24 hours following the conviction. And there were multiple reports of hate crimes against Black servicemen and motorists and store clerks. The threat of change seems to bring the racists out of the shadows, and we are paying attention. We have been educated by the racist ex-president who spent four years in the White House; now we know what to look for.

In addition to police violence, there were 48 mass shootings in March, (*Gun Violence Archive*) which means there were four or more victims killed in each shooting. On some days, there was more than one mass shooting in America—in spas, homes, grocery stores, schools, churches and synagogues, and on the streets.

Most of the semi-automatic rifles and handguns the killers used were legally purchased despite previous police encounters. There are few limits to the violence we allow in this country and our extreme Supreme Court is debating even those. Is anarchy an acceptable price to pay for personal freedom? When taken to extremes, aren't they one and the same?

APRIL 28, 2021

	CASES	DEATHS	DAILY NEW	DAILY DEATHS
WORLD:	149,611,800	3,149,100	912,451	16,081
US:	2,257,610	573,951	52,605	712
INDIA:	18,376,400	204,832	379,308	3,645

When comparing "excess deaths" during the past one hundred years in the US, researchers found that there were more in 2020 than at any time during the past century...more than during the 1918 flu pandemic. And we are nowhere near the end of this pandemic; the death toll of the COVID virus will be historic, especially the global toll now being tallied by researchers around the world.

Infections and death are already historic in India. They are out of wood to burn bodies in Delhi, so they cut down trees that line the streets and shade the city parks. Family members wait hours for a turn to throw their beloved on the public pyre with a prayer. There is no other choice. Those who die at home are not counted, so it is reasonable to multiply the daily toll by a factor of ten or twenty—or as some say—by a factor of thirty.

Some scientists propose that the South African and California mutations have combined—called a "double mutant"—and are responsible for the second wave in India, in addition to new variants that have not yet been identified but are considered inevitable given so much transmission. The borders of India remain closed, flights to and from India have been canceled, and oxygen is the new currency.

Just today the vaccine makers in India have announced higher prices for vaccination in the mostly private hospitals for people with money. One wonders how international contributions will be distributed in India…likely from the top down given the priorities of most profit-driven governments.

Last year, during the first wave in India, they set up quarantine centers for migrant workers who were suddenly told to go home. During this second wave there are no restrictions or support for the millions returning to their villages. It is estimated that the daily infection rate in India will rise to half a million in the next month. Once again, the common good suffers while profits are counted.

MAY 3, 2021

The 2020 Summer Olympics in Japan were postponed last year due to the pandemic, but officials have insisted the Olympics can be held safely this year. Nearly 70% of the Japanese public has soured on the idea of holding the games during the pandemic since they are now in a fourth wave and only two percent of Japanese adults have been vaccinated.

However, leaders have insisted that the games go forward and have instituted several mitigation efforts: international spectators have been banned, the athletes will be tested every day, and competitors will return home as soon as their event is finished. But even with strict safety protocols in place, eight members of the Olympic torch relay team have already been infected. The 2021 Summer Olympics will start in July despite common sense and basic science.

Vaccine nationalism and toxic competition continue to hamper efforts to vaccinate the world. Rich nations are reserving their supply for internal use and poor nations are begging for a fair share. Some nations refuse to use vaccines from Russia and China because of a rushed process resulting in a low 60% efficacy. Russia and China use propaganda to disparage the mRNA vaccines developed by Pfizer and Moderna in the US despite 94% effectiveness. But even with good vaccines, the variants have dashed our hope of herd immunity anytime soon because we cannot vaccinate fast enough to stop mutations.

India is begging for hospital supplies and vaccines, and the world is responding with ventilators, PPE, oxygen and vaccine components; unfortunately, no vaccines will be available until the end of the month due to manufacturing failures in India, the world's premier vaccine center. COVID is sweeping the nation because the president of India held political rallies for his re-election campaign and sanctioned religious gatherings for a million of the faithful last month instead of preparing for a second wave. He was warned; he was also re-elected.

Brazil is also asking for help, but the world is not responding with the same enthusiasm due to the bullying and bravado of their president who continues to downplay the virus and ignore the consequences. There is talk of impeachment, but this will provide little comfort to those who still suffer and die by the thousands in Brazil due to his failures.

MAY 7, 2021

I could write about the booming US economy—with recent stimulus spending and impressive vaccination rates—but it is difficult to revel in our success while thousands in India commit the bodies of mothers and fathers and sisters and brothers and sons and daughters to the flame.

In pre-pandemic India, cremations happened in private and were concluded when an urn of ash was delivered to those still grieving at home. In the post-pandemic India, loved ones kiss a shrouded corpse goodbye while wood is piled on a public fire; they wear protective gear and watch as flames consume the body.

In this post-pandemic world, death cannot be hidden, cannot be confined to the hospitals and the mortuaries and the crematoriums; death from COVID is not a private affair. The funeral pyres in India are featured on every front page across the globe. Their suffering is illuminated by pyramids of flame and captured by journalists who record war-like scenes in real time.

We cannot look away while the fires burn since no one is out of danger...not yet. Even areas with steady vaccination rates are returning to lockdown; leaders are closing schools and restaurants and gyms for another few weeks because infections continue to surge. In our race between variants and vaccines, the variants seem to be winning. When we let down our guard, the virus always finds a way... always.

MAY 10, 2021

During the past decade the world has made great progress fighting poverty and in some places—including India—reduced the rate from a quarter to a tenth of the population using government programs and manufacturing jobs. But when manufacturing shut down during the pandemic, those gains were lost. And the India variant—B.1.167—continues to spread beyond the eastern borders of India to neighboring countries who are also at risk of plunging the gainfully employed back into poverty with required lockdowns.

Nepal has reported a 57% increase in infections even as the climbing season begins on Everest. Those infected are evacuated from the mountain but efforts to contain the spread will have limited effect due to close contact among climbers. In Cambodia, a very sudden and strict lockdown has left residents without enough food to survive while stuck at home. In Bangladesh factories are shut down and people have no income and no government support to buy essentials.

The opposite problem exists in the US where vaccinations have slowed the spread. Lockdowns are being lifted in most states and the hospitality industry is desperately trying to fill jobs for restaurant and hotel workers in advance of the summer season.

There are some who say that generous unemployment benefits are convincing workers to stay at home and nearly two dozen Republican governors are now refusing federal unemployment funds as a result. But others suggest that wages are too low, that jobs without benefits are less appealing, that priorities have changed for workers who spent a year at home thinking about their lives.

Again, I wonder what change the current pandemic might bring and it seems economic fairness is near the top. Working parents are tired of living in poverty while new billionaires are minted daily; they are tired of minimum-wage jobs with no benefits, tired of struggling to pay childcare and rent after working multiple jobs, tired of being one repair bill or hospital visit away from bankruptcy.

President Biden is focused on uplifting the living standards of American workers and his approval rating is 63%. It seems that "trickle-down economics" has finally run its course after forty-five years of brainwashing. People have realized that those at the top do not create jobs with their tax cuts; they purchase unimaginable luxury and political power. We see, once again, that time to think can have a big impact on the status quo, an unexpected pandemic benefit that has been consistent throughout the ages. When half the workers died during the Black Plague, the serfs who remained successfully bargained for more rights and actual wages. The poor finally had time to think...leading to centuries of progress.

MAY 17, 2021

	Cases	Deaths	Daily new	Daily deaths
World:	163,608,200	3,387,900	519,721	9,847
US:	33,020,322	586,765	32,032	613

While we were flying for the first time in fifteen months, the CDC announced that masks were no longer needed indoors or outdoors for fully vaccinated Americans...except on airplanes, trains, and where required by state law. The problem is that only 36.7% of Americans are fully vaccinated. The CDC made no recommendations regarding the unvaccinated except they should continue to wear masks.

Since there is no official certificate for receiving the vaccine and no penalty for refusing, we now have an "honor system" with the unvaccinated...with those who downplay the virus and refuse the vaccine and prolong the pandemic for all of us with their foolish demands for personal freedom.

As usual, I see no honor among those who have no interest in the common good; there is no honor for those who work against herd immunity in America. We will continue to suffer hundreds of deaths a day from a disease that could be stopped with a simple shot in the arm.

The rest of the world is no better behaved. Leaders in Japan still insist the Summer Olympics should go forward despite an overwhelming public outcry against the games and an underwhelming vaccination rate that still hovers around 2%. The entire medical community in Japan has joined the protest to no avail.

Meanwhile, India still suffers a catastrophic second wave caused by leaders who encouraged crowded elections and religious gatherings for millions of civilians who had no protection from the virus and limited healthcare to fight the disease. Nearly a thousand doctors in India have died from the virus in just four months; fifty died yesterday. And like a scene from *War of the Worlds*, hundreds of bodies float down the Ganges River because there are too many bodies to cremate.

The global COVAX vaccination program is stalled due to a lack of funds; millions of doses India promised could not be produced due to their own catastrophe. The US has offered twenty million doses, and other countries are stepping up including China and Russia, but it is a piecemeal effort defined by politics.

Politics will not stop the fourth variant from sweeping the world. India's B.1.617 strain has now spread to forty-four countries including the African continent which is on the verge of a crisis. Vaccines are effective but in the global race between vaccines and variants, the variants are winning because there is no collective will to vaccinate the world.

Now is the time to consider the potential benefit of a world government. Only a vested world government could have saved us from the absolute ravages of human fear and greed during a global pandemic.

MAY 29, 2021

	CASES	DEATHS	DAILY NEW	DAILY DEATHS
WORLD:	169,905,523	3,531,788	512,446	11,313
US:	33,267,937	593,920	11,590	338
INDIA:	27,894,800	325,972	194,953	3,815

The daily average of infections in the US hovers around 20,000 with the death rate from COVID falling to around five hundred souls per day, the lowest rate in fourteen months. These numbers represent a significant change due to the efficacy of our vaccines.

During the two weeks we spent in Colorado—together for the first time since Christmas—we wore masks when entering an indoor public space and on public transportation, but removed the masks nearly everywhere once seated. Even the new president greeted the press corps without a mask for the first time this week. "If you are vaccinated, take off your mask and smile!" Biden said.

The psychology of emerging from a pandemic is interesting to this retired counselor. Some of us are so hungry to gather again it was like flipping a switch—we decided to trust the vaccine and fully engage. Others emerge more tentatively after a year alone, frailer and more frightened; they have adjusted to loneliness so life beyond their cocoon seems overwhelming. Gun sales and anxiety rates are at record highs and there have been more than two hundred mass shootings in America in the first quarter of 2021. Some people have no remaining patience.

Regardless, this will be America's Reunion Summer. All the campgrounds and hotels are full; it is difficult to find lodging in nearly every summer vacation hotspot. The National Parks are over capacity and turning away the hordes of vacationers desperate to get out of the house.

And soon, we will begin to count the cost of our pandemic failure: How many children lost parents or were abused by parents who became desperate and lost control; how many bankruptcies and suicides and drug overdoses happened behind closed doors—the deaths of despair that result when we fail to protect the common good.

And how will we change as a result? Will a twenty-first century renaissance follow the 2020 pandemic?

JUNE 9, 2021

In the confusing early months of the pandemic many dismissed the theory that the coronavirus was caused by a security breach at a Wuhan virology lab, but we recently learned that three scientists who worked at the lab were admitted to the hospital in November 2019 with pneumonia-like symptoms. Was this a coincidence?

The medical records of these three workers have been sealed by Chinese officials who continue to insist that the Wuhan animal market located a block from the lab was the source of a "natural" virus… which is a reasonable theory but one they have failed to prove.

Seeking to exploit pandemic fear, the ex-president often spoke of "the China virus" or "Wuhan virus" leading to an explosion of hate crimes against Asian Americans and a corresponding reluctance for those with a more humanitarian bent to even consider the accusation.

But the global death and poverty caused by the virus deserves a full investigation of its origin, and the truth might never be known if China continues to protect its political reputation at the expense of scientific knowledge.

To combat ethnocentric designations, the WHO now refers to the variants with Greek letters starting with alpha, (beta, gamma, delta, epsilon). The variant discovered in India and now found on every continent has been designated "Delta." The Delta variant strikes fear in the heart of epidemiologists because it is fifty percent more contagious than all the previous variants, a possible catastrophe that requires a robust global response.

With 62% of eligible Americans having at least one vaccine we are ahead of the race between the vaccines and the variants, but the rest of the world is still far behind. With a goal of two billion shots by the end of the year, the WHO is begging for help. The US has promised 500 million doses and the global fund to purchase vaccine has grown to nearly two billion dollars, but there are eight billion souls on this planet. This is not the robust response required to stop the pandemic. Global events need a global response…there is no other way. We need a world government, or at least a coalition with teeth.

JUNE 15, 2021

	CASES	DEATHS	DAILY NEW	DAILY DEATHS
WORLD:	176,625,742	3,522,369	378,028	10,818
US:	33,452,993	599,875	13,452	341

The first state to issue a stay-at-home order was California on March 19, 2020, and it will lift all restrictions as of today. There will be no limits on gathering, no mandates for mask wearing, and schools will fully open in the fall. New York state will follow suit tomorrow.

President Joe Biden's goal of having 70% of Americans vaccinated by July 4th—Independence Day—will be reached in Democratic states but not in the fifteen Republican states that have vaccinated less than half their residents with one dose to date. In Mississippi and Alabama, it will take another year to reach 70% at the current pace.

The anti-vaxxers seem to be reaching mass hysteria within their social media groups. A delusional physician—testifying before the Ohio state assembly—tried to demonstrate how the vaccine "magnetizes" people by placing a spoon on various parts of her body…which promptly fell off. You can't make this stuff up…oh wait, they do.

For example, there is a VAERS (Vaccine Adverse Event Reporting System) data site to track any death of any person receiving any vaccine for any reason…designed to spot trends. If a person with high blood pressure died of a heart attack a month after a vaccine the death is reported on the site. Anti-vaxxers use the data to prove that vaccines cause death—lots of death—assuming without proof that everyone who dies after receiving a vaccine was killed by it. To date 300 million doses have been administered and three people have died directly due to the vaccine according to the CDC.

In Japan, they have reached a fourteen-percent vaccination rate, which is steadily rising. While the Olympic trials are conducted around the world, public opinion is shifting. The dedication and skill these athletes exemplify is uplifting at a time when we desperately need heroes. It is hard for me to stop watching the trials, with the spins and flips and laps of record-breaking athletes. The Olympics are always a celebration of what human beings can physically accomplish, but this year it is also a reminder that the virus has not won, not yet. We can still compete.

JUNE 21, 2021

There were two articles in *The New York Times* this week that examine the changes in how American workers have been influenced by the pandemic. The first theory called YOLO (you only live once) proposes that 40% of workers are contemplating not returning to their pre-pandemic jobs because of working conditions that include long commutes, long hours, inadequate health care or sick leave or childcare. It appears that having time for contemplation changes how you think about time.

The second article by David Brooks suggests that devastating events lead to innovation, and this is certainly evident by how many people are in the process of renegotiating their living environments and working relationships. White-collar workers are moving out of the cities in record numbers and those who do stay require additional perks such as co-working spaces in apartment buildings and flexible hours from employers. Blue-collar workers are returning to school and some employers are offering to pay.

And while outlandish election fraud claims—fueled by the ex-president—continue to motivate Trump's most ardent supporters, many voters seem ready to move on and there is hope that progress can outpace the politics of grievance in the not-so-distant future.

The unvaccinated are suing employers who require vaccines with arguments about personal rights and state-sponsored medical terror but their petitions to the courts are falling flat. They now account for most of the deaths from COVID-19 and still believe unproven claims of vaccine risks circulating like a virus on their carefully cultivated media feeds.

Regardless, the US is approaching Biden's 70% vaccination goal and there is every indication that the antibody protection will extend to the Delta variant now sweeping the world. Only four Democratic states still have restrictions, including Oregon where we are one percent short of our 70% goal. Unfortunately, most of the Republican states still rely on the "hope and a prayer" pandemic plan and have vaccination rates well below the goal.

JUNE 30, 2021

	Cases	Deaths	Daily new	Daily deaths
World:	182,193,387	3,946,837	371,413	7,882
US:	33,638,620	604,502	13,683	283

Only the vaccinated are winning the race with the variants; the unvaccinated accounted for 99% of the deaths from COVID in the US this month. The "wait and see" attitude of those who try to outguess science has been a deadly gamble. The entire country has lifted restrictions and will celebrate the July 4 holiday by crowding together, so hospitalization and death rates will likely inch up by the end of July.

The Delta variant that swept through India during April and May has proved to be nearly 60% more transmissible and highly virulent and has now circled the globe at warp speed. Just this month, ninety-five countries and all fifty US states have reported a growing threat from the Delta strain. Countries that were slow to order vaccines due to indolence or poverty are scrambling to vaccinate populations that are more at risk from the new wave. Sydney, Australia has locked down for the first time while cities in Russia, Africa, and Europe all report new restrictions due to the Delta variant.

The New York Times has estimated that pandemic death is underreported in thirty-five countries, especially in India where hundreds of thousands of deaths have not been counted. More alarming is the fact that the current wave in South America is three times worse than India's wave; the healthcare systems in Argentina and Columbia and Brazil are collapsing amid an overwhelming surge of infection.

Meanwhile, the Pacific Northwest enters week two of a heat wave that has sent temperatures soaring nearly thirty degrees above normal from Canada to California. Records are shattering, bridges and roads are melting, and hundreds are dead from the heat. The "heat dome" is slowly moving east, leaving drought and death and fire in its wake…and a new respect for the destructive power of climate change. The fire season is off to an early start and fire refugees will soon replace heat refugees at convention centers.

And still, as we emerge from isolation our joy is evident. We recognize each other without our masks and hug without fear. We accept dinner invitations and attend public events. We make plans despite a dawning realization that COVID will not go away anytime soon…not until the world is fully vaccinated. Maybe not ever.

July 15, 2021

	Cases	**Deaths**	**Daily new**	**Daily deaths**
World:	**188,932,826**	**4,065,896**	**546,987**	**8,001**
US:	**33,967,870**	**607,704**	**35,561**	**250**

The fourth wave is upon us. Missouri is one of a handful of states where hospitals have more COVID patients now than during any surge in the past fifteen months. Healthcare workers are asking for field hospitals to handle the overflow.

The Delta variant is winning the race because rejecting vaccination has become a badge of loyalty for Trump's base, and the conservative media is using misinformation to raise revenue. Vaccination rates directly mirror the election results and the former president's supporters are paying the ultimate price for their loyalty: Nearly all the COVID deaths this month have been among the unvaccinated.

Cases are rising in all fifty states, primarily among people in their twenties, thirties and forties, since 80% of seniors have already been vaccinated. Children under twelve are still not eligible but those twelve to eighteen can get the shot if their parents approve. In Tennessee, the public health director was fired for reminding the public that those fourteen and older can legally make their own healthcare decisions.

The hysteria regarding the danger of vaccines becomes more dystopian and deadly each day. In fact, the political party to which White males belong is a better indicator of longevity than every other measure. On average, all of us lost 1.5 years of life expectancy during the pandemic, the longest decline in the US since WWII.

The January 6 insurrectionists continue to be identified in social media posts mostly due to the selfies they took and distributed to document their insane euphoria after busting through the windows and doors of the Capitol. More than five hundred have been arrested and charged; today the first was sentenced to eight months in a federal prison. The FBI is aided by a civilian network called Sedition Hunters—online sleuths who help match images from the insurrection to faces on social media sites.

A flurry of books exposing the deranged and dangerous thinking of our ex-president have been published and will serve as a foundation for the historical indictment of his one-term presidency. These books are all bestsellers.

The organization that bears Trump's name is under indictment for tax fraud—among other crimes—but it is the historical record that will ultimately hold him and his administration accountable—especially those trying to retain support of the base by doubling down on the lies: The insurrectionists were just tourists! The 2020 presidential election was stolen! The ex-president will be reinstated next month!

Party leaders still make pilgrimages to Trump's New Jersey compound to receive a blessing for the 2022 midterms. The stolen election lie has become the litmus test for viable Republican candidates due to the alternative reality of their party leader—the one who lost by seven million votes in the last election. "It was stolen!" he says to anyone who will listen. The emperor has no clothes but the parade goes on.

Part Six: Delta Strikes

July 29—September 11, 2021

JULY 29, 2021

	Cases	Deaths	Daily new	Daily deaths
World:	198,612,607	4,228,860	648,048	9,359
US:	35,038,975	613,151	102,975	582

Last week I became a grandmother for the first time. Under normal circumstances, I would wind this journal down just as the next generation springs forth, but complacency has allowed the virus to mutate and multiply so rapidly that infections have increased tenfold in four weeks. Delta is many times more contagious and spreads like chickenpox; the viral load can be a thousand times greater than the original Alpha virus. The "war is changing," according to the CDC, and only half the nation is vaccinated. Delta is responsible for nearly 90% of all new infections. The pandemic is not over.

Wallowa County is a COVID hot zone due to the Whisky Festival held in Pendleton on July 10. We now have ten cases a day, and the surrounding rural counties report dozens—and sometimes a hundred—new infections daily among the unvaccinated. There are rodeos and music festivals and state fairs in full swing all over our great nation. South Dakota is expecting 700,000 riders at the Sturgis motorcycle rally starting next week.

In June we were down to 10,000 daily cases and in July there are 100,000. The COVID careful have resumed wearing masks indoors but too many others throw caution to the wind and crowd together without masks or vaccines.

Texas and Florida have more daily cases than they did pre-vaccine due to the efforts of their governors—Abbott and De Santis—to court favor with the Republican base. These leaders have signed executive orders banning all mask mandates citing the anti-health doctrine of personal choice; they refuse to encourage vaccines.

America is a rich nation with abundant resources and citizens with too little common sense, people who are easily influenced by false Facebook narratives. Vaccines are expiring in pharmacies while the unvaccinated fall seriously ill and eventually plead for the shot. But the option to vaccinate often ends once Delta grabs hold so they text heartbreaking regrets from a hospital bed and apologize with their final breath. Despite these public confessions, conservatives still protest masks and mandates on social media platforms flooded with misinformation.

The unvaccinated complain about being second-class citizens and the vaccinated are increasingly angry. After lockdowns and quarantines and economic devastation, after a fleeting hope that we might finally emerge with the help of vaccines, we find ourselves facing another surge and wondering why personal freedom trumps the common good. Don't people realize that children cannot be vaccinated yet and remain at risk?

Over 44,000 children are currently fighting COVID in pediatric hospitals in states with the lowest vaccination rates per capita; hundreds of children have died. Now parents face the agonizing choice between keeping their children safe at home or sending them back to school next month.

No amount of pleading has increased our vaccination rate, but fear is beginning to work. Those who decided to "wait and see" now wonder if they have waited too long…and the clock is ticking. Public health officials have warned that infection is all but certain for the unvaccinated because the Delta variant is determined to find them… has evolved in order to find them. We are currently losing the race between vaccines and variants. Delta is winning.

AUGUST 10, 2021

US records the most daily infections in eight months: 164,225

Oregon is the third state to implement a statewide mask mandate—universal masking indoors regardless of vaccination status—due to an unprecedented rise in COVID infections and hospitalizations and deaths. All Oregon state employees are required to get vaccinated; everyone in the US military is required to get vaccinated; those in colleges, in retail, in major league sports teams are all required to get vaccinated due to the rapid and uncontrolled spread of the Delta variant. The idea of personal choice during a pandemic is dying a painful death.

Now we know that the infection rate of transmission—the R0—of the original (Alpha) virus was between two and three; one infected person spread the virus to two or three other people. The R0 of the Delta variant is between six and seven which has given rise to an exponential increase in infections; one infected person can spread the virus to thirty-six people in two degrees of contact. (1 x 6 x 6 = 36) and in three degrees of contact (I hang with her indoors; then she hangs with him) the number of likely infections rises to 216.

There were 700,000 new COVID infections in the US last week and 96,000 of the infected were young children…double the rate from the week before. The pediatric ICUs are filling up across the nation and many are dying.

And still the governors from Florida and Texas are competing for Trump's blessing by banning masks and refusing vaccine mandates even though these two states account for nearly half the new infections. Parents and businesses are bringing lawsuits by the dozens to stop the personal freedom madness the Republican politicians have unleashed upon the nation.

Keith and I will not travel to Denver to visit our first grandchild as planned. We strongly suggested they keep the baby in a strict bubble until the danger passes, the paternal grandparents in Rhode Island also agreed and canceled their visit.

In our small resort town, the infection rate is soaring, and a vacation here no longer seems as safe and inviting as it did just a month ago. Reservations are being canceled and the stores and restaurants and bars usually packed this time of year are suddenly half full. The unvaccinated will be responsible for a new round of economic destruction as well as a rising death toll, and we all pay the price for their ignorance and selfishness and greed.

Most of us are heartsick to be going through another surge when we were so close to normal, but COVID deniers and election deniers and vaccine deniers are obstinate and oblivious, enthralled by the MAGA cult of personality. Will they ever wake up?

AUGUST 13, 2021

With the apex of the new surge expected around September 7th, the unvaccinated will soon have missed the window to protect themselves with a two-dose vaccine since it requires six weeks to complete. The COVID cautious are stocked up and hunkered down until this extremely high surge is behind us. The rates of infection and hospitalization are setting new records for the entire pandemic; deaths are still low due to the successful campaign to vaccinate 80% of older adults, but now younger adults are filling the ICU's and dying a preventable death…including children. Unlike the original Alpha, the

Delta variant does not discriminate by age...any vulnerable person will do.

Infection rates in the south—especially in Florida and Louisiana—are now higher than anywhere in the world even though the US has an ample supply of vaccine soon to expire in the pharmacies. Once again, the US accounts for 25% of global cases with only five percent of the population.

There are marches and protests and fistfights over mask mandates in public schools; doctors are being threatened for providing public health information at school board meetings. It feels like half the country has gone mad (again) and indeed, Trump continues to rally his base against public health even though they are now sick and dying as well as crazy with anger.

Behind the scenes and the headlines, some COVID skeptics are facing reality. The daughter of a friend texted me this afternoon, wondering if I was vaccinated. She knew I was—of course—but wanted to start a conversation. For eighteen months she ignored public health advice and resented the mandates. But she needs the vaccine to vacation abroad and was struggling with the decision. After a brief exchange of facts presented with empathy, she decided to get the Johnson & Johnson one-shot vaccine this afternoon. Please don't tell anyone, she asked, especially her MAGA mother.

We are not the same country we were five years ago. Tribalism is the weapon of choice for dictators—to divide and conquer—and the neofascist we elected in 2016 and defeated in 2020 is still trying to destroy the US democracy, to retain power and profit from chaos. The hundreds of millions Trump has raised with his "Stop the Steal" campaign represents a political threat without precedent in our nation's history—his base is enthralled and still believes the election was stolen despite an absolute lack of evidence. The ex-president's soul is in danger: To knowingly spread deadly lies for personal gain constitutes iniquity.

AUGUST 17, 2021

	Cases	Deaths	Daily new	Daily deaths
World:	208,942,754	4,387,195	812,138	11,428
US:	37,114,590	623,423	204,003	1,528

The pandemic continues to mirror the progress of humanity: those with resources do not value the very thing that those without resources desperately need; inequality flourishes amid record profits; the self-righteous attack those who serve the common good.

And we learn—once again—that a pint will never hold a quart, that you can lead someone to water but you cannot make them drink, that two steps forward is usually followed by one push back. This is the dance of human evolution, the pattern of progress.

The silent majority who are guided by science are being pushed back by the vocal minority who find an emotional release from protesting; despite facts, they promote false arguments because it feels good. This familiar dance between progress and fear—good and evil—has defined civilization throughout our history and once again there are severe consequences. Death from this virus can now be contained but instead the rate is climbing; our children are caught in the crossfire between the science of public health and the self-service of personal freedom.

The one step back we now endure will be an object lesson for the future. Personal freedom cannot supersede the common good without everyone paying a price…in personal freedom. Freedom is a shared ideal not a personal right. Tens of thousands of children are now being quarantined because a few parents demanded the freedom to choose if their children will wear a mask in school.

Eventually both freedom and progress will be defined in the crucible of the common good but for now the minority rules…and we take a step back.

AUGUST 24, 2021

	Cases	Deaths	Daily new	Daily deaths
World:	213,518,161	4,457,007	665,108	10,110
US:	38,106,086	630,440	153,296	1,318

Israel was the first nation to vaccinate against COVID using the Pfizer shot, aggressively securing and delivering the vaccine starting in December 2020. A few months later, 80% of the population age twelve and up were fully vaccinated; by mid-June there was not a single case of COVID recorded in Israel and all restrictions ended. Israelis celebrated and traveled… and brought the Delta variant home with them.

Two months later they again reached peak infection rates with 10,000 daily cases and hospitals filled with COVID patients. Nearly five hundred have died. After another aggressive booster campaign, cases are now falling but the evidence points to a waning protection from mRNA vaccines in six to eight months possibly due to the variants; everyone will need a booster shot.

The WHO chair pleads with rich nations for a booster delay, citing the need for vaccines among poor nations with low vaccination rates. Only a global campaign can control the pandemic, but the healthcare industry must commit to the project. The world needs vaccine factories on every continent with vaccine formulas readily available in the public domain. Unfortunately, the global capitalists who fund such endeavors are not yet willing to share formulas or fortunes.

At home, the chair of the National Institutes of Health suggests that the Delta variant is causing a new pandemic, replacing the Alpha with a variant that is two times faster than the original—faster at transmission, onset of symptoms, serious illness, and death. The CDC just published a study showing unvaccinated people are twenty-nine times more likely to end up in the hospital with a serious infection. With ninety million unvaccinated Americans, Delta is surging everywhere including Wallowa County—a red-hot zone with infection rates as high as those in the Deep South. Cancellations and closures and quarantines are announced by the hour in major cities, and many establishments are requiring proof-of-vaccination to enter. There is a booming market for fake vaccination cards however, so even people who have no interest in the common good can benefit from those who do.

The FDA finally approved the Pfizer vaccine for everyone sixteen and older, which gives cover to companies who want to mandate vaccines for workers. No more "experimental drug" excuses. Vaccination rates are improving slowly and there is hope for a run on the Pfizer vaccine soon.

But the heartbreaking battle against mask mandates in public schools is where the real damage is being done. If children of the unvaccinated come to school unmasked it does no good for other children and teachers and school staff to wear masks...without universal vaccines, the Delta wins and so does minority rule. Florida school boards and parents are fighting the anti-mask orders with civil disobedience; half the public schools have mask mandates despite the governor's threat to cut funding.

Trump held a rally in Alabama last weekend and casually suggested people should get vaccinated. He was booed by his Republican base, so his immediate follow-up was "But of course, you still have your freedoms. And who knows if the vaccines work?" It is not purely partisan opinion that links COVID denial with support for the ex-president. County comparisons all show a consistent correlation between low vaccination rates and high Republican votes in the 2020 presidential election, a beast of Trump's own making he can no longer tame.

There are seven unvaccinated pregnant women on ventilators in Alabama fighting for the lives of their unborn children as well as their own. As a mother, I can imagine how these women agonized over the best way to protect their babies...but were misled by misinformation on conservative media sites. Where are the vocal right-to-life Republicans when we need them?

SEPTEMBER 2, 2021

It seems to me that the world is fighting two viruses at the same time: The COVID virus, which has already killed at least five million people, and the virus of vulture capitalism which has accelerated climate change in the pursuit of profit. To reach the apex of vulture capitalism, corporations have bought and sold political leaders, degraded the facts of science, and twisted the common good into an opposition party that conservatives seek to destroy; everyone needs an enemy.

The war is fought upon the battlefield of social issues where emotions are easily manipulated. What is good for the whole, this part is against. In the new conservative utopia, there will be no civil rights, no voting rights, no climate science, no gay rights, no women's rights, no racial equality, and no gun laws. In this new utopia, the new conservatives (neo-fascists) attack public health as a loyalty pledge for the (White male) base.

Unfortunately, those who adopted this agenda of opposition to progress are now consumed by the consequences along with everyone else. The harvest of greed—and power—is upon us.

In the past week, wildfires consumed thousands of acres and homes in the West due to unprecedented drought, high temperatures, and the destructive winds caused by climate change. In the South, hurricanes—now more frequent and more destructive—were followed by record rains creating flash floods that raced through neighborhoods. A million people have no power or gas in southern Louisiana; the poor are sweltering in homes destroyed by the storm. Hospitals once filled with unvaccinated COVID patients have been evacuated to neighboring states.

The same storm then moved to the Northeast and flooded New York City, where basement apartments became deathtraps after rain fell three inches an hour. Climate scientists tell us this is just the beginning.

The next generation will recognize the truth: Due to unfettered profit-taking and self-serving politics, the current generation allowed climate destruction; we were warned but did nothing. And still, we fiddle while the world burns.

SEPTEMBER 10, 2021

I have been documenting the pandemic for eighteen months, a year longer than planned. Tomorrow the nation commemorates the twentieth anniversary of the terrorist attack of September 11, 2001, the day we collectively realized that no amount of money can keep us safe. There was a transient unity in our shock, but fear has divided us in the two decades since.

Fear has become a community poison and continues to hold us back. The solution to the pandemic, one the US could have shared with the world, is difficult to implement even in our own homes and communities. One in every five hundred Americans has been infected with the virus and more of us have died these past months than during the entire 1918 pandemic, even though we have effective antiviral medications and an effective vaccine.

The pandemic has become a weapon in a political war fueled by misinformation and fear. Democracy itself is threatened by The Big Lie. Trump continues to hold fundraising rallies and still rejects the 2020 results nearly ten months after the election. He plans another run for the presidency in 2024.

SEPTEMBER 12, 2021

	CASES	DEATHS	DAILY NEW	DAILY DEATHS
WORLD:	**219,372,719**	**4,547,260**	**660,323**	**9,622**
US:	**39,626,789**	**644,633**	**176,941**	**2,937**

Last September, when there were 28,000 daily infections, schools closed to stop the spread and classes were moved online. Today there are 150,000 daily cases and children are back in the classroom. Unfortunately, children account for 26% of new infections, totaling 250,000 in the past week. There are 2,500 children in the hospital and tens of thousands being sent home to quarantine—with fewer online options for learning.

And still, there are anti-mask protests across the nation and here at home. Last week, Wallowa County protestors were pictured on the front page of the weekly paper encouraging parents to send their kids to school unmasked in violation of the Oregon governor's mandate. "Don't be sheep!" one speaker said.

Delta has created another dangerous surge in the pandemic, and 100,000 more people may die before this terrible year ends. I am reminded of the parable shared by pastors and priests about the dying man who wonders why God has abandoned him. When he reaches the pearly gates, he asks why his faith did not save him.

God replies (and I paraphrase): I created science to help you evolve beyond suffering, but you were focused on fear. I inspired doctors to help you stay safe, but you were filled with disdain. I even sent a new vaccine, but you turned away, demanding personal freedom. So yes, you are here of your own free will, another gift…although faith in my plan could have saved you.

We are sheep. We mask-up to protect the lambs.

Part Seven: The Fifth Wave

December 15, 2021—April 19, 2022

DECEMBER 15, 2021

	Cases	Deaths	Daily new	Daily deaths
World:	272,217,900	5,328,693	625,975	7,214
US:	50,346.987	801,037	121,188	1,302

My beloved brother, Don, died of pancreatic cancer in early October; he was diagnosed and dead within six weeks. He was our bubble-mate, and we were careful not to risk any COVID exposure during the past eighteen months. Little did we know that the pandemic we feared would not be what killed him; the pandemic afforded eighteen months of quality time while the cancer quietly spread. Our time together in lock-down was a blessing.

We hoped for one final Christmas together, but his suffering ended quickly, and we join a million other American families who will miss a loved one at the holiday table this year. I took time off from writing to grieve.

In the three months since the last entry, another 150,000 Americans have died of the virus; most were unvaccinated and succumbed to the Delta variant that swept the nation starting mid-summer. Only

60% have been fully vaccinated in the US and 50% worldwide, with poorer nations still left behind in the vaccine race.

Refusal to receive the vaccine due to misinformation is a global problem facilitated by the digital information age. It's easy to fall down the online rabbit hole of misinformation promoted by friends and enemies in equal measure. The anti-science tribe has never been more robust.

Consequently, the hospitals are overflowing with unvaccinated COVID patients while general surgery patients wait for a bed. Exhausted healthcare workers are leaving the field in record numbers.

And now a new variant—Omicron—is sweeping the world, causing new lockdowns and travel restrictions and fears of another deadly surge. The CDC has issued Do Not Travel warnings at the highest level for eighty countries and counting.

But people are still traveling, both domestically and internationally. Pandemic fatigue has created an insulating fog of denial and an accepting calm, especially now that full vaccination includes a booster shot. There is hope that boosters will keep Omicron at bay, but this variant—with thirty-plus sub-mutations—has evolved to overcome our defenses and now threatens the vaccinated and the unvaccinated alike; only a third vaccination offers enough protection.

This week the January 6 House Select Committee released evidence that proves there was an elaborate plan to overthrow the results of the last presidential election. The bi-partisan congressional committee has acquired and presented evidence—PowerPoint presentations, email chains, text messages—and is holding the leaders of the coup in contempt of Congress because they refuse to answer subpoenas. The Department of Justice has indicted over six hundred insurrectionists for storming the Capitol and many will spend the holiday in jail.

Extreme weather continues to plague the country. This week there were a series of unprecedented December tornadoes that killed sixty-seven workers at a candle factory in Kentucky. One especially strong twister was on the ground for 212 miles and traveled across four states. There has been record snow and wind and rain in the past few days.

Our plus-one family is grateful to be gathering for the holiday again. Last Christmas our children isolated together and then traveled home in one vehicle. This Christmas they decided to travel separately and use at-home COVID tests to rule out infection once they get here. We are all triple-vaccinated so the risk is minimal, but since the baby cannot receive a vaccine yet, we will also isolate for five days before she arrives to add another layer of protection.

JANUARY 6, 2022

The pandemic rages on with the highest daily infection rate ever recorded in the US—704,369—and the results ripple through every aspect of American life.

Finally, on the one year anniversary of the January 6 Insurrection, President Biden delivered a blunt speech denouncing the "Big Lie" of a stolen election—a lie that continues to rally Trump's MAGA believers and threatens democracy. Biden finally accused Trump of an inability to accept defeat and said, "he holds a dagger at the throat of America."

There is an abundance of recently published books, magazine and newspaper articles, interviews with politicians and political historians, all warning that our beloved democracy may not survive if there is a repeat insurrection following the 2024 presidential election. Fascism continues to attract a third of the nation and spreads like a second deadly virus.

The Omicron variant has quickly traveled the world. There is no country spared, no haven for the weary. Businesses are closing again, including cruise ships, sporting events, indoor dining, theater, college classes…anywhere people gather. The CDC and WHO expect daily infection rates here and abroad in the millions for the next few weeks—and then the surge will pass.

The silver lining is that this variant causes less serious lung damage leading to fewer hospitalizations and deaths. But Omicron is many times more infectious and has a shorter incubation period than the powerful Delta strain. Experts warn that this variant might infect fifty percent of the global population before the surge ends.

As we enter year three, we clearly see how the pandemic has shifted our perception of human behavior and injured our mental health. Pre-pandemic scenes of people packed tightly together still send a momentary shock through us. A new fear of proximity to the other has invaded our consciousness. Images of people in a crowded elevator or market or concert trigger our fight-or-flight response: proximity means danger.

Women have always understood this feeling—it leads them to cross the street when unknown men walk the same path at night. But now this feeling rises for men as well, when random people simply stand too close or pass by without a mask or stroll down the same aisle in the grocery store, coughing. It is a conditioned fear response that will linger long after the virus loses its battle with the human immune system; fear of the other will be a legacy of COVID.

JANUARY 14TH, 2022

	Cases	Deaths	Daily new	Daily deaths
World:	323,794,053	5,528,933	3,536,828	8,890
US:	65,049,258	848,542	924,343	2,951

The pandemic continues to create hardship for American families and businesses. With nearly a million cases per day reported by testing centers, and an unknown number of positive home tests, the new variant has brought the country to its knees again.

A severe shortage of tests feels like déjà vu. Home tests are all sold out, so people wait in long lines for lab tests to see if a holiday exposure requires a five-day isolation. They must produce a negative test to return to work and most have no sick leave. But new rules from the CDC allow asymptomatic workers with a positive test to return after a five-day isolation period (instead of fourteen) and asymptomatic healthcare workers who test positive can return to work immediately because hospitals are overwhelmed.

Unfortunately, schools and daycare centers and cruise ships are closing without notice because of staffing shortages. In some industries, thirty percent of the staff have called in sick since Christmas. The domino effect of staff shortages leads to supply-chain issues and empty shelves. Another round of business closures is at hand—this time without stimulus aid. The eviction moratorium is set to expire; student loan payments resume in May; unemployment benefits have run out. And there are a million new cases of COVID a day…that we know of.

The WHO has predicted that half of Europe will be infected with the new variant in a month; the CDC says everyone in the US will eventually get COVID.

And still, the US Supreme Court overruled President Biden's vaccine mandate for businesses, writing in a six-to-three opinion that OSHA overstepped its mandate by requiring employers to vaccinate workers. They did uphold the requirement for healthcare workers to be vaccinated, but the five-to-four decision is too late for the overwhelmed hospital system suffering from an exodus of staff due to illness and burnout.

More than half the nation's hospitals have less than ten percent capacity in the ICU. Hospitals are filled with more COVID patients than since the pandemic began and most are unvaccinated. The only good news is that the Omicron variant strikes hard and fast and recedes the same way; infection rates are already going down.

JANUARY 26, 2022

	Cases	Deaths	Daily new	Daily deaths
World:	381,675,145	5,686,787	3,262,391	10,234
US:	75,285,898	889,522	424,077	3,576

Eight billion doses of the vaccine have been administered worldwide, with 77% immunized in high-income countries. The US fully vaccinated rate is 64%, which is one of the lowest rates among wealthy countries. There were 3,576 deaths reported in the US from COVID today.

The twice-impeached, fully disgraced ex-president Trump, who planned a coup to steal a second term, held a rally over the weekend in Texas and promised pardons for the January 6 insurrectionists AND a civil war if he was re-elected president in 2024. His comeback "Save America" rallies are part of a pseudo campaign designed to further radicalize the fringe fascists of the Republican party and build his bank account. Supporters have contributed $122 million to Trump's political fund as of this month.

His supporters are also attacking school boards and teachers over Critical Race Theory—which is the actual history of any person or group who is not a White heterosexual Christian—and banning books in public schools. Teachers are leaving public education in droves and joining the "Great Resignation" along with childcare workers and healthcare workers and anyone else who has been trying to serve the public during the pandemic. The National Guard has been called up to replace the missing teachers.

Tens of millions of American workers voluntarily quit their jobs in 2021. Again, I am reminded of the Black Plague in the Middle Ages that decimated the serfs and eventually led to the Renaissance, a rebirth of philosophy and art and literature between the 14th and 17th centuries. The common people finally had enough time and money to improve their minds.

Faced with the difficulties of working during this pandemic—with no sick leave and poor wages and no benefits—workers are once again refusing the crumbs left by the corporations and the CEOs who make 10,000 times more per hour than those who supply the physical labor. The ten richest billionaires in the world (all White men) doubled their wealth during the pandemic. This points to an obscene corruption of capitalism, a profit fetish at the expense of the people.

Meanwhile, the infection rate for the Omicron variant is starting to fall sharply although hospitalizations and deaths are higher than ever. There will be a million Americans dead from COVID sometime this spring and according to post vaccination studies, eighty percent of the current deaths are in counties Trump won in 2020. Unvaccinated Republicans are dying from COVID at a rate five times higher than Democrats. I am sorry for the pain these families must endure.

There are rumblings that a second Omicron variant (BA.2) is circulating and may be even more transmissible than BA.1. In the meantime, the tide of sentiment regarding mitigation efforts seems to be turning towards accepting more risk. Is it time for the fully-vaccinated to resume normal activities?

Every household in the US is eligible to receive four free at-home COVID tests in the mail with a simple sign-up on the US Postal Service website. The first tests are arriving this week, just as the fifth wave begins to recede. Once again, we are behind the curve.

There have been dozens of natural disasters in the two years of this journal but none as dramatic as the undersea volcano that erupted near the island of Tonga in the South Pacific on January 15. The explosion—with the power of five hundred atomic bombs—sent a tsunami all the way to the Oregon coast and an ash cloud twenty-four miles into the air. The satellite photos are stunning but there was grave concern for the citizens of Tonga, who could not be reached for several days. Although there was significant structural damage, only three casualties have been reported so far.

FEBRUARY 4, 2022

The 2022 Winter Olympics opened today in Beijing, China with a zero tolerance COVID policy. Chinese workers have quarantined within the Olympic village complex for two months and there are few spectators allowed. Several top-ranked athletes have withdrawn due to positive COVID tests and are now housed in the quarantine quarters. In addition to being seriously disappointed, they complain of intolerable accommodations and inedible food, which feels like punishment.

The zero-COVID policy extends throughout this communist country of 1.4 billion people. An entire province of four million was locked down for two weeks recently when a cluster of fifty cases was discovered. There are reports of a "no mercy" attitude as well, with death from other emergencies and sudden hunger considered a necessary sacrifice to contain the virus. As usual, hosting the Olympics shines a global light on the successes and failures of the home nation.

Johns Hopkins released a chart ranking death per million from COVID in each country through February 2, 2022, with Brazil first, followed by the US, Mexico, the EU, and South America holding the next four spots. China's communist regime comes in last and *appears* able to enforce public health protocols with very few deaths. At what price, many ask? The contrast between American individuality and Chinese control in pandemic management could not be more stark, although public health organizations report having no data from China since April 2020. This communist country is keeping secrets from the world.

Experts are pondering the cause of such high cases in the top four countries, and some have settled on "trust in government" as the best indicator of a people's willingness to choose public health over personal freedom. It feels like a failure to be sandwiched between Brazil and Mexico; it feels like our own unique kind of corruption to have the highest healthcare costs in the world and the worst outcomes of any wealthy nation. Our place on the chart—and in history—has been secured by our singular focus on profit at the expense of public health. So exceptional, we are.

FEBRUARY 11, 2022

	Cases	Deaths	Daily new	Daily deaths
World:	408,135,287	5,801,293	2,412,283	10,806
US:	77,531,295	917,140	187,325	2,474

The far-right movement was unleashed in 2016 when a reality television host and talented grifter named Donald Trump won the presidency by stoking fear of the others and "freedom" from the constraints of civilization. The balance between self-control and selfishness was undone, privilege was hailed as patriotism, and prejudice was normalized. Half the voters became enthralled.

The pandemic became the perfect foil for the fight against civil constraint. Once the base had been primed by endless rallies and angry speeches urging people to "stand up" to elites and leaders, the pivot to anti-masks and anti-lockdowns and anti-vaccines was easy.

The far-right media took up the call and people organized online. After losing re-election by seven million votes, Trump continued to control the base by attacking democracy directly with the Big Lie of a stolen election. He gathered and incited a mob at the US capitol on January 6, 2021, and then watched the violent insurrection on a television in the White House cafeteria; he said nothing while his MAGA followers set up gallows and threatened to hang Vice President Mike Pence, who was certifying the vote.

Civilization is constrained—governed—by law for a reason. There is no other way to control our innate animal nature: we are hungry by design and must decide between what we want for ourselves and what is fair to others on a daily basis...and sometimes hourly. Fairness is often elusive.

As predicted, the Omicron variant reached unimaginable heights in just a few weeks and then fell equally fast. The reported cases do not accurately reflect how many were infected because people finally have access to home tests, and the illness from Omicron seems to be less severe—which bodes well for herd immunity. Nearly everyone has either been vaccinated or infected...or both.

The new Omicron sub-variant, BA.2 has yet to make a splash, so most states have announced an end to mask mandates starting next month. Once again, people are hopeful that the pandemic is over... but COVID is a wily creature that adapts to every possible weakness.

Infection rates are down nearly seventy percent, hospitalizations by fifty percent, and the death rate is inching lower. Still, 15,000 people are dying of COVID each week. California is the first state to consider an endemic response as opposed to a pandemic response: Clusters will be investigated and traced, and equipment will be stockpiled, but there will be few mandates. We hope the worst is over; we know there are no guarantees.

FEBRUARY 24, 2022

Despite two months of high-level talks to defuse tensions, and just days after the Winter Olympics ended, Russia invaded the sovereign nation of Ukraine today, attacking from three sides with tanks, missiles, bombs and bullets. Russia's goal is to reclaim the largest client state of the failed Soviet empire, to force a "war of conquest" upon a very determined democracy in eastern Europe.

Really, this is a continuation of the global conflict between democracy and autocracy, what Biden called "a sinister vision for the future of our world," a vision embraced by Russian president Putin, who has poisoned or imprisoned his challengers for the past twenty years to consolidate and expand his power.

Autocracy is winning according to the Bertelsmann Transformation Index (BTI) that tracks the rise and fall of democracy worldwide. The current score in developing countries is Democracy 67 and Autocracy 70, the first time in the fifteen-year history of the index that autocracy has become dominant in the world.

True to form, Trump and his sycophants praised Putin, calling him a "genius" for infiltrating Ukrainian borders with Russian separatists and then invading to "protect" them. Since the US presidential election in 2016, there has been a pro-autocracy drumbeat on right-wing media, including public support for strongmen, that boggles the mind: Do you really want to lose your voice, your vote, your personal freedom?

It is ironic that these same people demand freedom to refuse pandemic mandates but think nothing of denying freedom to others;

these same "patriots" wave the American flag while they storm the Capitol during an insurrection against the American Constitution; these same public figures swear an oath to democracy on one hand and support autocracy on the other…for power and profit.

Both World Wars in the twentieth century started in Eastern Europe after assassination and invasion; both required a significant sacrifice to push back against autocrats—men like Hitler and Mussolini and Stalin who believed themselves to be the embodiment of an entire nation.

Hitler declared "I am Germany!" in 1939 before he invaded and imprisoned and exterminated his neighbors, before his war to make Germany great again killed 85 million people, before he was defeated by the Allies and retreated to a bunker to commit suicide in disgrace.

Putin believes he can "make the motherland great again" by attacking his neighbors and shocking the world. We have faced bullies before and have defeated them—a never-ending challenge—but not without a surprising amount of destruction. There is a high price to pay whenever a powerful bully seeks to make "his" country great again. But ultimately, bullies destroy…they do not build.

A hundred years after World War I and the Spanish flu, we again face dual threats from a brutal war amid a tenacious pandemic. Have we learned nothing from history?

FEBRUARY 28, 2022

	CASES	DEATHS	DAILY NEW	DAILY DEATHS
WORLD:	436,939,086	5,955,034	1,559,979	9,310
US:	78,942,537	948,855	64,276	1,855

The entire world has been shocked by Russia's invasion of Ukraine. Since the Russian president destroyed a free press, his misinformation campaign convinced older, more isolated Russians that invasion was justified, but some Russians risk arrest and imprisonment to protest in the streets. The Russian president's propaganda is quite contrived: that Ukraine was never a sovereign nation, that the leaders of Ukraine are Nazis (even though their president is Jewish), that the people of Ukraine have pleaded for help. Lies, all.

As expected, the Russian president has underestimated the strength of the Ukrainian desire for independence and democracy; he has underestimated the unifying effect of his attack upon a nation seeking NATO protection; he believed that strongmen rising in failing democracies would support his challenge. He was wrong.

The people of Ukraine are fighting back. Although nearly 500,000 women and children and elderly are evacuating to neighboring nations—refugees who have left homes and schools and lives behind—most able-bodied citizens have taken up arms in a civilian brigade and partnered with the regular militia in defense of their nation.

The courage of the new Ukrainian president has impressed the world. "I need ammunition, not a ride," he declared when offers to evacuate poured in. He knows he is the number one target for elimination should Russia succeed. He continues to inspire Ukrainians, and even ex-pats living abroad are returning to join their children and parents on the front lines. Their willingness to fight for freedom is another miscalculation by the Russian president and serves as a needed reminder to the world: Democracy is worth defending with your life.

As the global resistance builds, the Russian president appears unhinged and responds by putting his nuclear forces on high alert. In turn, a coalition of nations has crippled his economy with the most devastating economic sanctions on record. Russia cannot buy and sell goods in the global economy. Even Switzerland has frozen deposits for the first time in history. Russian rubles have lost 25% of value overnight; the Russians stock market was closed today.

The International Olympic Committee has recommended that no Russian athletes be allowed to compete in international events; the cyber hackers are waging war on Russian websites; social media platforms have suspended Russian commerce on their sites; FedEx and UPS have suspended deliveries to and from Russia…the list goes on.

Suddenly, much of the world is standing up to a bully, is facing down an autocrat, is firmly invested on the side of democracy. Ukraine will suffer greatly at the hands of these invaders and the world is watching. In the twenty-first century, how can aggression against a sovereign nation be worth economic collapse, to say nothing of the ethical and moral questions that come to mind when watching entire families flee bombed and burning buildings.

The pandemic is taking a back seat to the war in Ukraine. But across the world the numbers of cases and hospitalizations and deaths have fallen dramatically and the new variant, while present, is struggling to find purchase among the vaccinated and unvaccinated alike. The CDC has relaxed recommendations for masking; protests are becoming moot.

Perhaps the courage we see in Ukraine will inspire all of us to rejoin the world.

MARCH 2, 2022

President Biden gave his first State of the Union address last night, beginning with the war in Ukraine and ending with the progress on COVID. For the first time since 2017 both sides of the aisle stood in solidarity to condemn Russia and to affirm progress in the pandemic. The relief we felt as Americans was stunning according to all the reviews and articles released today. There was no blame, no shame, no divide-and-conquer rhetoric that effectively set us upon each other during the past four years. It was a humble and unifying speech to reassure the nation. It feels like a sea change.

The news about COVID continues to be positive. Recently the CDC announced the results of comprehensive tests to detect COVID in blood samples and estimated that 140 million Americans contracted the virus during the past two years, which is around 44% of the population. Since 65% of us are fully vaccinated, our protection against COVID has improved considerably.

In addition to the end of mask mandates, there will be no more contact tracing. The new strategy announced by President Biden is called "test and treat" which guarantees an immediate and free antiviral treatment onsite when someone tests positive for COVID. Antivirals are very effective at limiting serious illness and millions have been ordered by the federal government to distribute to local pharmacies and clinics. Such good news.

At the same time, our hearts are breaking for the carnage in Ukraine. The capital is surrounded, and the Russians are firing missiles at neighborhoods and government buildings and historical sites in order to crush the spirit of the people. It is not working. In less than a week the Russian president has managed to destroy his economy and isolate his country from the rest of the civilized world; he has provided an object lesson for Western democracies that freedom requires strong alliances and a common defense.

There is no world government coming to the aid of Ukraine, not yet. But suddenly we see a turning point: people are choosing freedom and becoming responsible for its defense with their lives and their livelihoods. Even the giants of capitalism are choosing to support Ukraine against the invaders. Democracies cannot let a dictator destroy the common good. Hopefully, never again. Idealistic, I know, but hope springs eternal.

Another war for the soul of the world has begun. General Omar Bradley, commander of US Army Troops during World War II, troops that defeated Hitler and his Nazi regime, summed up his fears a few years after that war ended:

"The world has achieved brilliance without wisdom, power without conscience. Ours is a world of nuclear giants and ethical infants. We know more about war than we know about peace, more about killing than we know about living."

MARCH 9, 2022

Nearly 775 individuals have been arrested for participation in the January 6 insurrection and the first jury trial ended with a conviction, leading many of the accused to consider a plea bargain instead of a trial.

The Supreme Court upheld the January 6 Congressional Committee's right to subpoena phone and email records for the investigation into how the coup attempt was planned and executed. The Supreme Court also ruled that Fox News must defend itself against charges of libel in a pair of billion-dollar lawsuits brought by two voting-machine companies that were repeatedly accused of facilitating voter fraud on the network's daily news programs.

Trump still pretends he won, picking sycophants to run for Republican seats all over the nation, flying to fundraisers in his private jet, spewing word salad on conservative media outlets, pretending he does not approve of Putin after publicly praising him as a genius. Our "mad king" makes no sense and neither does his friend in Russia.

It does make sense, however, to view these power-hungry males as vestiges of our animal nature, posturing and attacking to retain status. We cannot consider ourselves civilized while allowing world leaders to acquire power through violence and corruption. Humanity cannot progress until the rule of law and the common good are the primary goals of leadership.

The Russian president is a perfect example of the danger of absolute power. While tightening his grip on the country for twenty-three years, he engaged in unethical and immoral acts with impunity and was eventually corrupted. Some say the pandemic further affected his state of mind. His COVID isolation was extreme and his protocols apparent in the photos where he positioned himself twenty feet away from every other person in the room, a symbolic scene in which he is literally untouchable.

And now, the entire country—spanning eleven times zones—must endure global isolation as the West imposes unprecedented economic sanctions and hundreds of corporations withdraw. A second Iron Curtain is descending upon the largest nation in the world.

In stark contrast, the president of Ukraine has shown true leadership and has rallied the democratic world in defense of freedom with an eloquent voice and effective defense against an invading dictator who seeks to expand his own standing in history. The president of Ukraine, Volodymyr Zelenskyy, speaks to the world, reminding us of our "Never Again" pledge after the last World War when German Nazis initiated a war of conquest that eventually led to eighty-five million deaths including the extermination of six million Jews.

Now, world leaders must choose between a global economy and personal power, between the rule of law and absolute control, between relative peace and World War III.

MARCH 17, 2022

	Cases	Deaths	Daily New	Daily Deaths
World:	**465,862,971**	**6,064,173**	**1,784,859**	**5,106**
US:	**79,568,137**	**968,663**	**30,550**	**1,224**

For two years, Hong Kong has been a model of virus control with a "zero COVID" policy that included testing and contact tracing and isolation for those exposed including a strict two-week quarantine. While the rest of the world was dealing with surges from Alpha and Delta and Omicron, the people in Hong Kong went about their daily lives as if they were immune; there were no mask mandates and little incentive to risk vaccines that were considered dangerous and unnecessary especially by the elders.

During the past few weeks, a surge of BA.2—with an infection rate (RO) of ten (one person can infect ten)—has overwhelmed Hong Kong's COVID defenses. With seven million people packed into a country occupying a scant 435 miles, population density is the fourth highest in the world; it is estimated that half of the population has been infected by the highly-transmissible variant this year. The healthcare system is stressed, and the death rate is currently the highest in the world; they have run out of room for the dead.

Other Asian countries with strict COVID policies and low infection rates are also being hit hard by the BA.2 sub variant including South Korea—with a new daily record of 600,000 cases—Vietnam, Thailand, Singapore, and China, where millions are subjected to lockdowns when COVID is detected. In some countries, early success is now a curse.

BA.2 is making headway in the UK and Europe as well, and accounts for 25% of the COVID cases in the US. With 65% of the US fully vaccinated and immunity from high-infection rates in the past few months, there is hope that the BA.2 variant will not lead to more hospitalization and death. But historically, a surge in Europe precedes a surge in the US by just a few weeks. Only 60% of our seniors are protected by boosters, which means nearly twenty-eight million may have waning immunity a year after the first dose. Moderna has requested FDA approval for a fourth booster for those over the age of sixty-five, and Pfizer for all those over eighteen.

The pandemic has exacted a greater toll on the world than reported. It is estimated that the number of deaths related to COVID is three times higher than official counts according to studies published in *The Lancet* that found 18.2 million more deaths above the global average in 2020 and 2021.

There is additional evidence that the coronavirus did originate in a seafood market in Wuhan, China. The working theory is that caged animals infected shoppers with a transmissible virus in November 2019, but China refused to acknowledge human-to-human transmission until January 20, 2020, which allowed travelers to spread it around the world in less than three months.

Highly contagious variants are still spreading three years later, unfazed by other deadly events in the world. Like most living organisms at war, they respond to threats by retreating and re-arming and then attacking again.

March 22, 2022

Republicans only voted for relief funds for Ukraine after funds for COVID were removed from the bill. In the face of continuing variants, the US has exhausted the money set aside for testing, vaccinations and treatment. We can only hope our defenses hold.

The support for Ukraine both at home and abroad is stunning. Ukrainians from all over the world are returning to fight while young Russians are leaving their country by the tens of thousands, anti-war refugees who are ashamed of Russian aggression. Their parents and grandparents blindly believe Putin and approve of his anti-Nazi "special military operation." Russia is starkly divided while Ukraine is intensely united.

Leaders from thirty NATO nations are meeting in Brussels, an alliance of democratic nations that Trump tried to destroy at the urging of the Russian president. But the 1949 alliance between Democratic nations is stronger now than ever, a strategic partnership originally designed to defend against ongoing Soviet aggression after the Second World War.

In southeast Ukraine, the Russian army is bombing Mariupol to create a southern corridor from Crimea—which the Russians seized in 2014—to the Russia border. The 200,000 residents who were not able to flee have no water or food or electricity or places to hide since most of the buildings have been destroyed. Anguished loved ones accuse the Russian soldiers of genocide; war crimes have been committed.

In southwest Ukraine, a flotilla of warships lines the horizon west of the port city of Odessa on the shore of the Black Sea where they launch missiles to weaken the western defenses, but they have failed to seize the city.

The Russian president expected a quick victory and now looks desperate. The world wonders if he is desperate enough to use chemical or biological or nuclear weapons. More than 10,000 Russian soldiers have died in the past four weeks, and nearly 30,000 more are either wounded, or captured, or missing. The soldiers who return home will know the truth about those who did not return. How long will their mothers be silent?

Autocracy rises when people are hungry but lies cannot feed them. Closed systems feed on themselves, and the ones who create them will eventually devour their own. In the absence of democracy—and the benefit of group wisdom—the common good is sacrificed and the ones who rule become criminals, people who act with no moral compass. Once again, we see the truth: power corrupts, and absolute power corrupts absolutely. Autocracy is a failed system that leads to delusions and death and destruction. Democracy must be defended, always, everywhere in the world.

MARCH 29, 2022

	CASES	DEATHS	DAILY NEW	DAILY DEATHS
WORLD:	**485,187,402**	**6,131,933**	**1,586,738**	**4,806**
US:	**79,920,438**	**977,179**	**29,253**	**716**

Life in the US is getting back to normal for most of us. This month I traveled to the East Coast to help Rachel move to Providence, Rhode Island to start a much better job at Brown University, and this weekend I attended an outdoor birthday party with fifty of my closest friends, people I have not seen for nearly three years. The joy of reuniting was palpable; people hugged each other fiercely and huddled around the bonfire to exchange stories about all that has happened since March 2020. I was struck by how familiar their stories were: They stayed in the county, worked from home in a shared office, enjoyed the outdoors but were isolated from friends; almost all celebrated births and mourned deaths and worried about catching COVID.

The FDA approved a second booster for those over fifty, so more protection is on the way. The Omicron BA.2 variant is now dominant in the US, but the results of an active spring break have yet to be determined; another few weeks will tell the tale. There are few reserves left for caution so most of us wear masks only when required in healthcare facilities and airports. It feels liberating.

Michael is traveling to Poland to help open a refugee center. An informal coalition of nonprofit groups in Denver and Poland have agreed to help with the project titled "Palaces for People." They hope to house some of the two million Ukrainians who have escaped to Poland in the past four weeks by turning destination wedding venues into turnkey refugee centers. A Jewish non-profit in Poland will help settle the first group of refugees outside of Warsaw.

Hannah is halfway through medical school, mostly spent alone in her bedroom on a computer. She will be home this weekend with no questions asked—no testing or quarantines even though she spent the past week with her boyfriend in California studying for board exams. We feel almost guilty looking back at what we required during the past two years. She asks if there were any special measures needed this visit and was surprised when we quickly said, "Nothing at all."

APRIL 11, 2022

For the first time in a month, COVID cases in the US are rising, especially among the elite in the nation's capital where nearly one hundred cases were reported after six hundred high-ranking politicians attended a party unmasked. Very few experienced severe illnesses since most have been vaccinated.

The BA.2 variant is still causing havoc in China where millions languish in strict lockdown with little access to food. People are summarily marched off to quarantine centers if they test positive or are imprisoned at work with few basic comforts. There have been small protests, a rare sight in China.

Now that a second booster—a fourth shot—is recommended and available in the US, there is a renewed sense of security. Hospital rates and death rates continue to decline across the nation. The light at the end of the COVID tunnel shines brighter every day even though the darkness of war lies heavy upon the world.

April 19, 2022

	Cases	Deaths	Daily new	Daily deaths
World:	**505,875,744**	**6,201,998**	**726,984**	**2,641**
US:	**80,645,527**	**987,999**	**41,989**	**410**

Although a "zero COVID" policy worked well in China during the first two years of the pandemic, all 25 million people in Shanghai—the world's largest city—have endured three weeks of strict quarantine. Drones roam the city broadcasting the message: "Control your soul's desire for freedom." People have no food, medicine is running low, and those with medical emergencies are still denied care, causing unnecessary death.

Chinese authorities have shuttered the factories and the financial district, causing a ripple effect through the global economy. The totalitarian government failed to produce a viable vaccine, and then failed to vaccinate the population. The variants have found an inviting home.

The world is under threat from forces unwilling or unable to progress. Democracy is still in its infancy and requires a global village to reach maturity; those suffering from the alternative—autocracy—will someday demand democracy, proving the soul does have an uncontrollable desire for freedom.

In the meantime, we witness the rise of poorly-educated workers who rightly complain that inequality has rendered them slaves. The poor have been abandoned by politicians, while billionaires spend obscene profits to ensure there are no laws restricting obscene profits. The workers will revolt.

Despite this imbalance, people still live and love and grow. Humans are designed for growth, and eventually—after fear and greed and war have failed—the higher good will prevail.

Since progress requires an elevated perspective, it no longer feels productive for me to get lost in the weeds of daily conflict. The goal of this journal was to document the pandemic for my grandchildren, and it seems the end is near—or at least the beginning of the end here at home.

To the grandchildren for whom this journal is intended: In you, progress resides. You are well loved, even by those you only know vicariously, through a shared history.

Love travels through time…can you feel it?

Epilogue

AUGUST 2024

TOTALS AS OF APRIL 13, 2024:
WORLD INFECTIONS: 704,753,890 / DEATHS RECORDED: 7,010,681
US INFECTIONS: 111,820,08 / DEATHS RECORDED: 1,219,487

COVID is not over, but it no longer feels like a deadly threat. Last week I had an eighth Covid booster during a routine visit with my primary care physician. The last time I wore a mask was on a plane to Hawaii in March, but I was maskless the entire flight home. Those who feel sick stay in bed for a few days as normal, but there is no talk of isolation or quarantine. When we see someone in a surgical mask, we assume their immune system is compromised.

Since states no longer collect daily COVID data, public health organizations are not tracking in-depth information—infection and death counts from the April 13, 2024, are the most recent from Worldometers.com. To date, the US has suffered 17% of all recorded global deaths from COVID with just 5% of world population. At the height of the pandemic, we suffered 25% of global deaths, but that number went down when our vaccination rate went up.

However, if our number of deaths was directly proportional to our share of global population, we would have 350,534 deaths instead of 1.2 million currently recorded. We also know that researchers who looked at excess global deaths from years 2020–2022 found 25-35 million more deaths than normal during the COVID years, lonely deaths that were never counted due to limited public health resources and willful ignorance.

Another way to see the scale of the US death toll from COVID is to consider this: In all the wars America has fought since 1775 the total number of soldiers who died was 1.3 million, just a hundred thousand more than the 1.2 million *recorded* deaths from COVID in two years. The coronavirus was not just a little flu; it was a global pandemic just as lethal to those in the United States as 250 years of war.

There are other medical consequences from the pandemic that are considered a mystery: an increase of unusual cancers in young people and a surge of more than thirteen viral and bacterial infectious diseases and respiratory ailments above global normal, including colds, measles and tuberculosis according to reporting by *Bloomberg News* (June 14, 2024) which analyzed data from sixty news organizations and public health agencies. People around the world are suffering from physical illness at ten times pre-pandemic levels due to a likely combination of factors including an end to isolation, a lower vaccination rate, a mistrust of healthcare professionals and issues with the immune system caused by the virus. The pandemic made the world much sicker than usual.

There are social consequences as well. School children are behind a year in all subjects at every grade level, and some have not returned to school for unknown reasons. Suicide rates have increased due to loss and grief and continued isolation. People seem to have less emotional resiliency and are often less tolerant of others leading to arguments, fights, and murder.

Economic loss—especially among small business owners and ethnic minorities—has led to food and housing insecurity, as well as an unprecedented increase in inequality. The poor have become much poorer, and the rich are much, much, much richer. The pandemic made the world less resilient, less tolerant, and much less fair to those without privilege.

The world is also more dangerous. As of this writing, Russians are still bombing Ukraine in a proxy war between authoritarians and those pledged to defend democracy in the West. Since ex-president Trump is a "friend" of the Russian president, MAGA followers in the House of Representatives have tried to stall military aid for Ukraine. And there are other serious lethal conflicts outside the scope of this journal.

Trump takes credit, as he should, for the six conservative justices on the Supreme Court who ended federal protection for abortion. As a result, women are denied treatment for difficult pregnancies or miscarriage management in red states, and the evangelicals are hard at work trying to deny all abortion and birth-control medication and in-vitro fertilization nationwide. Family doctors are leaving red states to avoid draconian laws; pregnant women are forced to give birth or die trying.

There have been a dozen similar high-stake rulings by the Supreme Court this session covering gun control, contraception, homelessness, January 6 incarcerations, and a handful more that will define life in America. The bias and corruption of at least two conservative Supreme Court justices has been confirmed by reports of partisan flags flying at vacation homes, lavish trips paid for by conservative billionaires, family involvement in the January 6 insurrection, slow-walking the question of presidential immunity to benefit the ex-president, and nonsensical rulings using "context" from the 1800's. Trump was correct when he stated he needed the ninth justice to retain the presidency. His 6-3 court has lost all credibility; Trump corrupts everything he touches.

And the court bias continues. Even though 1,500 insurrectionists have been charged and tried and found guilty in federal courts, the Supreme Court may use an obscure ruling to overturn the convictions and provide immunity for the ex-president's involvement in the

January 6 insurrection. America is suffering from minority rule, the result of structural flaws in our constitutional government that need to change if we are to survive. One person, one vote, no electors, and term limits for justices would be a good place to start. Oh, and no convicted felons in the White House.

We face authoritarian rule, climate change, emerging pandemics, armed gangs, escalating inequality, the threat of world war, and diminished compassion for others—for diversity. As a result, we have no choice: fair-minded Americans must respond or prepare for another century of destruction and death.

We know that truth and beauty and goodness travel through humanity quietly, without fanfare, an endowment of mind that resides within—a powerful weapon, ready and waiting. It is a good time for good people to rise and unleash the highly contagious virus of love; it is a perfect time for those who seek truth to stand against those who spread lies for personal profit.

I believe we grow in response to suffering, so from this perspective the future looks bright.